Nail Art

Nail Art

K-Sa-Ra

CHARTWELL
BOOKS, INC.

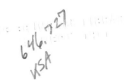

Published by Chartwell Books
A Division of Book Sales Inc.
114 Northfield Avenue
Edison, New Jersey 08837
USA

0-7858-1065-X

QUMNLAT

This book is published by
Oceana Books
6 Blundell Street
London N7 9BH

Project Manager: Rebecca Kingsley
Editor: Lyn Coutts
Design: Ray Barnett
Photographer: Paul Forrester
Picture Co-ordinator: Nancy Roberts

Manufactured in Singapore by Eray Scan Pte Ltd
Printed in Singapore by Star Standard Industries Pte Ltd

14.95

Contents

Introduction   6

Chapter 1   Polish secure Designs   17

Chapter 2   Stick-on Art   25

Chapter 3   Dream Transfers   33

Chapter 4   French Designs–a polished art   41

Chapter 5   Glitter Dust   49

Chapter 6   Embossed Designs   57

Chapter 7   Paint and Polish   65

Chapter 8   Hands-on Nail Art   73

Chapter 9   Foil Designs   81

Chapter 10   Airbrush Nail Art   89

Chapter 11   Nail Jewelry   97

Chapter 12   Pure Fantasy   103

Introduction

You may think that busy hands and concealed feet go unnoticed and their purpose purely practical, but you're wrong. The Chinese started reading hands in 5000 BC, and some psychoanalysts believe that the hands and feet are intimately connected to the psyche. So are you, by sitting on your hands to hide your nails, revealing something negative about your personality? In Far East Asian cultures, hand movements are a language for story-telling and love. The slow, measured, and graceful arm movements of Thai dancers, their natural nails hidden under long, curved talons, are sensuous and often erotic.

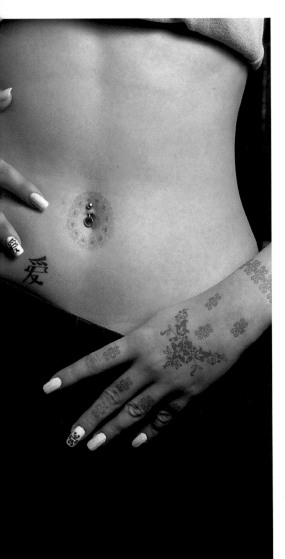

LEFT: Body decoration in all its forms is as old as humankind. For some it holds its traditional and symbolic meanings; for others it's a means of expressing and showing their individuality.

Richly-painted and adorned hands and nails are a symbol of wealth in Middle Eastern cultures. Mendhi markings painted with a henna dye are symbolic, but can be "read" like a book to reveal family and age. The toenails of harem women in Turkey were painted with henna to spell out love messages. Cleopatra, never one to miss a trick in the games of love or politics, painted her nails using vegetable or mineral dyes. The first nail-painting session–though a total accident–most probably involved both Mr and Mrs *Homo erectus* and iron oxide. When iron oxide, which has disinfectant, deodorizing, and protective properties, was smeared over their bodies, their nails would have taken up the stain and been tinted an attractive rust-red color.

While evidence aplenty exists to show that body decoration is as old as humankind and as natural, it has attracted some derision in modern times. "Painted ladies" was a euphemism for one of loose morals, and with the rise of puritan values in many religions in the West, the wearing of cosmetics was banned. In England, in the 1770s, the ban was justified on the basis that cosmetics were a way of entrapping a man into marriage.

But that is history, and today nail art in all its forms–from the understated to the over-the-top–is a star in its ascendancy. Since the days when car enamel and nail polish were one-and-the-same, technology and science have combined to create nail products of outstanding quality, finish, and color; the better ones fulfiling both sirens of fashion and the call for nail-friendly products. Experiments with nail polishes containing Kevlar–a substance used in the fibers of bullet-proof vests–would make the ultimate polish guaranteed to make weak nails rock-hard. Nail care and nail art go hand-in-hand.

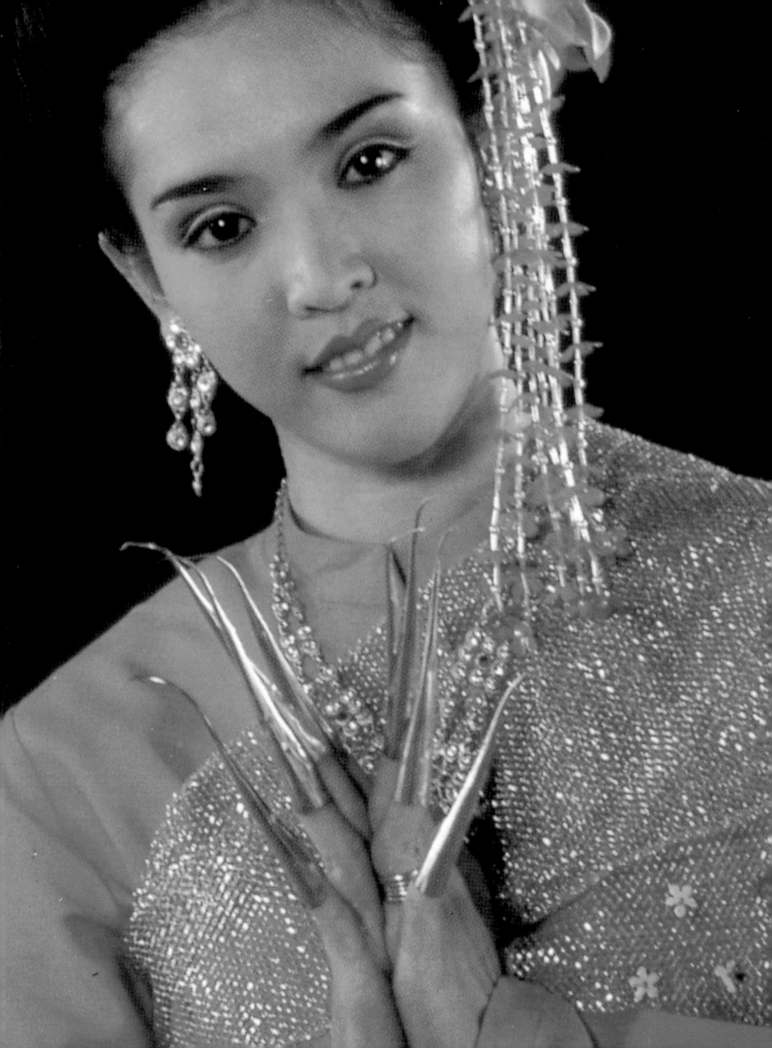

The shape of things

The shape of your natural nails will, in part, determine their length and how they are best polished and decorated to flatter. For square, triangular, or fan-shaped nails (narrow at the cuticle, wide at the nail tip), leave a narrow strip either side of the nail unpolished. Fan-shaped nails can be given the illusion of a more regular shape by leaving the half-moon unpainted. Avoid exaggerating narrow nails with stripes running the length of the nail.

A talented nail artist can do much to flatter your nails by suggesting suitable designs and colors. Should you decide to have nail extensions, then the whole spectrum of nail artistry is at your fingertips.

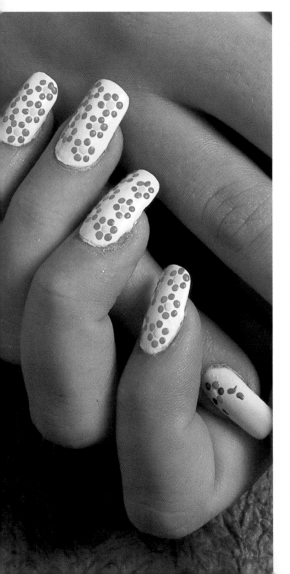

Colors, colors, and more colors

The number of nail polish colors grows every season, as do the types of finish. (A situation made more daunting as nail paints can be mixed to create any color you want.) Newer additions to the shelves include: metallic polish that is reminiscent of copper, brass, steel, or other polished metals; glow-in-the dark and in-your-face fluorescents and neons; and glitter polish, pigmented or clear, containing suspended dots or strands of glitter in one or many colors. No doubt, as nail art increases in popularity, the range of polish finishes will continue to blossom.

With all this choice, it would be comforting to know there were some rules about what color suits what, but there aren't.

The stereotype of "good girls wear pastels and bad girls wear red" just doesn't hold anymore. Pastels, once the domain of the young and brides, are worn by all; glitter and bright-lights colors are no longer just for parties, they also go to the office, gym and and on country walks; and the reds–once the only colors for sophisticated women– have been joined by purples, browns, greens, yellows, and oranges.

Feel the quality

There is a big difference between good and poor quality nail polish–and the difference is not necessarily the price. A good polish is easy to apply, has excellent adherence, and resists chipping. Its color is true, even, and has depth. With some poorer polishes, no matter how many layers are applied, the finish is never satisfactory and durability, poor.

Nail polish know-how

- The stainless steel ball in the bottle is to make mixing a uniform color easier.

- Store away from sunlight and heat, preferably in a refrigerator.

- Don't shake the bottle. Instead turn it upside-down and roll it between your hands to minimize the formation of air bubbles that accelerate drying-out.

- Buy small, rather than large, bottles of nail polish.

- Don't break a nail trying to open a nail polish. Instead, rub a little petroleum jelly around the neck of a new bottle.

LEFT: The quality of the nail polish is evident the moment you apply it. The color is uniform and deep, it coats completely, and looks spectacular.

RIGHT: There are no limits to the skills and imagination of a nail artist. Designs can range from cute hearts and flowers to the burlesque and bizarre.

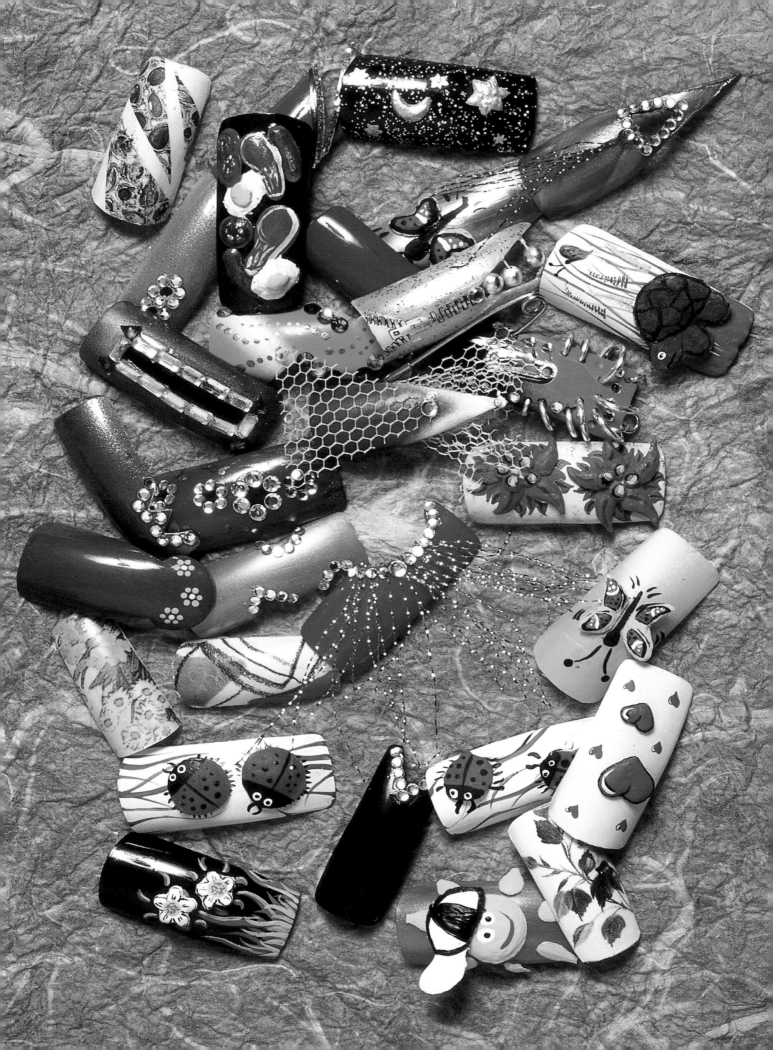

Glowing with health

Healthy nails are a sign of general good health. Therefore, what is good for you–a balanced diet and plenty of rest and exercise–is good for your nails. Genetics, though, does play its part, and having strong or brittle nails could be simply down to the genes you've inherited. If you're worried about the condition of your nails, and no amount of kindly treatment seems to remedy a problem, see a professionally-qualified nail technician. The scope of a nail technician's work extends well-beyond manicuring and polishing. Solutions and practical advice for a whole range of nail problems are literally at their fingertips.

The basic recipe for strong, vigorous nails is a balanced diet that consists of foods high in proteins (your nails are almost pure protein) and a cocktail of vitamins and minerals.

Vitamin A, calcium, and iodine strengthen nails, inhibit splitting, and promote growth. They can be found in varying amounts–and in the company of other beneficial nutrients–in butter and other diary products, fish and shellfish, fresh green vegetables (especially spinach or chard, broccoli, and

Nail doctor

Brittle nails–other than going out of your way to avoid contact with detergents (rubber gloves are a must) and extremes of temperature, wear your nails short (sometimes called the "sporty" length), buff them regularly, and use a quality nail hardener. As a matter of habit, always wear soft wool or leather gloves in cold weather.

Bruising or black marks–these will grow out naturally and usually result from hitting or trapping the nail.

Bump or dents–these are usually caused by inflicting rough treatment to the nail or by an illness. Even a short-term illness where your diet is affected and medicines prescribed, can affect nail strength and condition.

Flaking nails–avoid trimming with nail scissors as they can put unnecessary strain on the nail. Keep the nails short and use a nail strengthener.

Splitting nails–file the nails to a squarish shape so that the nail tips will better resist breaking. Applications of white iodine can

also help, along with wearing nail polish and a strengthener.

Stains–any number of things can stain the nail surface or behind the nail tip, and one of the kindest ways to remove the stain is with lemon juice. But to conceal the staining short-term, whiten behind the nail tip with the dampened tip of a white nail pencil. Staining caused by wearing strong-colored nail polish can be prevented by first applying a base coat.

Vertical grooves–this is one you can blame on your DNA and treatment is often a waste of time.

Weak nails–the root problem may be poor diet, but while the benefits of a major diet revamp take effect, apply a nail strengthener and rub in almond or olive oil nightly.

White marks–these are bubbles of air trapped between the nail bed and the nail plate, and they will grow out naturally. White marks can also be a side-effect of an illness.

If you are worried about the condition and health of your nails, seek professional help.

watercress), carrots, tomatoes, apricots, and cherries. Nail consistency is promoted by sulfur, which is present in cabbage, cucumber, and onions.

A biotin deficiency (biotin is a member of the vitamin B family) can be the cause of brittle nails.

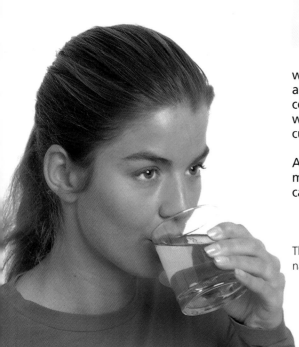

The secret of great-looking, healthy nails is a balanced diet.

Biotin-rich foods include eggs, peanut butter, wholegrain foods, and liver. The perfect between-meal snacks that can help to deter the formation of ridges and counter some of the effects of a serious illness are sunflower seeds, rye bread, and walnuts.

Any major beneficial changes in your diet will take about six months to show on your nails. If your diet is rounded there is no need to take supplements.

Nail cosmetics

Base coat–this provides a surface over which nail polish can be applied. It stops the nail from being stained by strong nail polish colors. Some base coats contain a nail hardening formula.

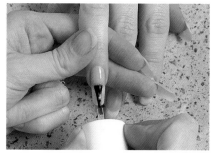

Apply a base coat everytime you polish your nails.

Cuticle conditioning cream–keeps the cuticles soft and easy to care for. A nail oil or almond oil can be used for the same purpose.

Cuticle remover–this loosens and lifts the cuticle off the nail plate. It can have a drying effect.

Emery boards–these are much kinder than metal files, whose use professionals advise against. They are available in different grades of coarseness, but unless your fingernails are extremely strong, opt for fine grades of emery.

Hand and nail moisturizing creams–there are any number on the market, but look for those containing a UV filter. A water-based emulsion cream is suitable for all-day use; use an emollient cream for overnight treatment.

Nail buffer–sometimes made of chamois leather, it is gently rubbed over the nail plate, often in conjunction with a buffer paste, to give nails a natural-looking shine.

Nail conditioner–there are many proprietary brands, but lemon juice, cider vinegar, or almond oil, applied daily are equally effective.

Nail extensions or tips–for many, these semi-permanent gel, fiberglass, acrylic, or silk miracles make nail glamor possible. Each type of extension requires a different application and removal procedure. The best advice is to have extensions done initially by a professional, so that your nail health can be checked and you can see what is involved.

Nail polish or varnish–see pages 8-9.

Nail polish remover–always use an acetone-free remover to prevent nails drying and becoming brittle.

Nail polish thinners–used to thin nail polish when it begins to dry in the bottle. Never use paint thinners or polish remover for this job.

Nail scissors–unnecessary if a manicure is carried out regularly, and only use when the nails are firm, not softened by warm water, otherwise splitting will occur.

Nail separators or pedi-pads–insert the soft foam ridges between the toes to make it easier to apply polish.

Nail strengtheners and hardeners–sometimes incorporated into a base or top coat, these serve the dual purpose of protecting the polish and making the nail more resistant to breaking. It is recommended that some stand-alone strengtheners or hardeners be used for only short periods, that only the nail tips should be painted, and that contact with the skin around the nail be avoided. Read the use and application instructions on the packaging carefully.

Oils–a few drops of almond, olive, or a prepared nail oil, rubbed nightly into the skin around the nail, will promote nail growth and strength. Smooth, uncracked skin around the nail and soft cuticles are bonus side-effects.

Orangewood sticks–used to push back softened cuticles and to clean behind nails. Nail technicians may sometimes use metal tools for manicures, but orangewood sticks are more forgiving in amateur hands.

Stick-on nails–these cover the entire nail and are secured using a glue or cement. Though different shapes and lengths are available, there will always be compromise about "fit" when using home-kits. Removing stick-on nails without the correct solvent, or wearing them too long, will leave the nail plate damaged. False nails are available in plain, colored, or decorated finishes; a "plain" nail must be finished with a nail polish. They are best used as a short-term measure to conceal a broken or badly-shaped nail, or for a special occasion.

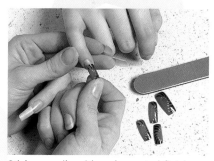

Stick-on nails with a decorated finish make nail art as easy as 1,2,3!

Top coat–applied over pigmented polish to give a smooth, shiny finish and to resist chipping. A top coat can be one or two coats of clear nail polish.

White nail pencil–wet the pencil tip and "color" behind the nail tip to conceal discoloration and to give a clean look. A nail bleach can also be used, but an application of lemon juice can be just as effective.

Nail art-the fun begins!

Great nail art can be created with just a few bottles of nail polish, a home-made stencil, and a thimbleful of rhinestones. But for those who want to take nail art to the limit, they may find the urge to accumulate the tools of the professional nail artist too hard to resist.

Acrylic nail paints (1)–water-based and non-toxic, these are used in varying dilutions for embossing, paint and polish designs, and airbrushing. They can be mixed together to create other colors. Also available are opalescent and neon nail paints.

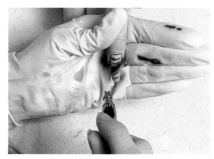

Airbrushing produces a distinctive and professional finish.

Airbrush (2)–used in conjunction with a compressor and regulator, the airbrush achieves spectacular results by spraying a fine mist of water-based paint under pressure onto the nail. The paints can be mixed to create a rainbow of colors, and they dry quickly. Prior to airbrushing, the nails are given two base coats; one to protect the nail, the other to provide a surface for airbrushing.

Art brush (3)–used to paint detailed pictures and designs on nails using acrylic paints. Try to buy the best quality, fine-tip brush you can afford.

"Color Shaper" tools–these are used to create textured designs on nails with nail art paint. The "Cup-round tool" dabs and

blends, the "Angle-chisel tool" is used for strokes and lines, and the "Taper-point tool" for spots, marble-effects and flowers.

Craft knife (4)–for cutting your own stencils from "Frisket" film or masking tape.

Cutter punch (5)–when placed on a sheet of "Frisket film" (clear, self-adhesive film bonded to a peel-off, backing sheet) and the top depressed, it cuts a stencil. There are many cutter punch designs available.

Decals and transfers (6)–there are two types: water-release and self-adhesive. Water-release designs are freed from their backing when dampened with water. The design, held on very thin, clear film, is then placed on the nail.
Self-adhesive designs are peeled off their backing sheet and positioned on the nail. Self-adhesive designs, though in some ways easier to use, are thicker and therefore more noticeable. There are scores of different patterns and images; with the most detailed being lace, snakeskin, and feather decals.

Embossing tool–used to create raised designs on the nail. The syringe is filled with a thick, acrylic nail paint and when the plunger is depressed, the paint is pushed out of the tip in a controlled way to create lines, dots, swirls, and patterns.

Fan brush (7)–the splayed hairs of this brush create sweeps of color across the nail. They are used in paint and polish designs.

Flatstones, rhinestones, diamond crystals, sequins, cabochons, and "Dazzells" (8)–these are secured by placing them, flat-side down, on wet nail polish.

Foils (9)–when rubbed onto a nail, partially or totally covered with foil adhesive, it leaves a multi-colored or metallic "coating" on the nail. Its effect cannot be replicated by other nail art techniques. Another form of foil leafing is used only on wet polish.

Glitter-dust (10)–when mixed on the tip of a brush with a special mixer liquid, glitter dust powder forms a dense and rich "polish," unlike any type of sparkle or glitter nail polish. Glitter dust comes in many colors and is easy to use.

Guide tapes (12)–self-adhesive, crescent- or chevron-shapes that make it easy to paint French polish designs.

Lace (13)–acts as stencil when held tightly over a nail. Most commonly used in conjunction with an airbrush.

Liner brush (21)–used in paint and polish nail art to paint thick lines and to cover "large" areas with paint.

Marbling tool (15)–use the ball-heads to blend layers of wet polish or paint on the nail to create a marbled-effect. Can also be used to make dots and swirls, and to position polish-secure decorations.

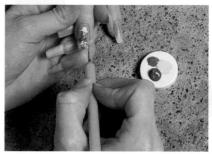

The marbling tool in action creating a paint and polish design.

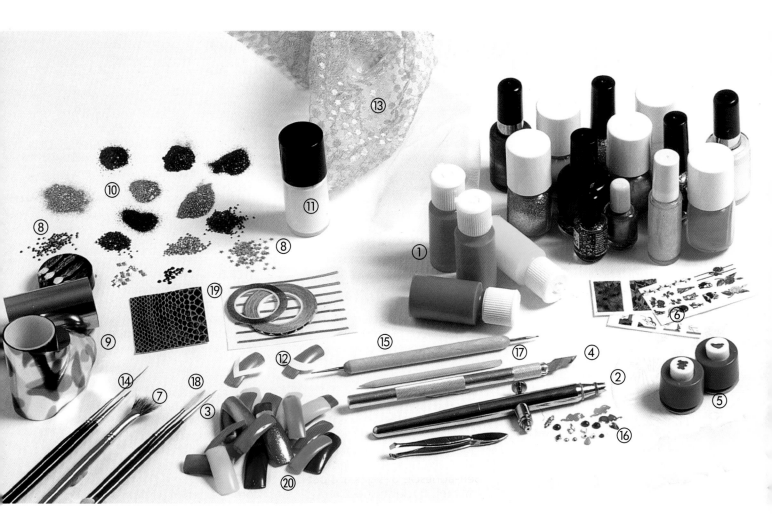

Nail adhesive glue–used to attach stick-on nails and some decorations to nails. Ask a nail technician to recommend the glue suitable for your purposes, but always follow the manufacturer's instructions.

Nail jewelry–once a small hole is drilled into a nail extension–never a natural nail–modest to dangling nail jewelry can be worn. Plated charms, beads, crystals, precious gems, and chain jewelry can be securely worn using these methods of attachment: a ring; a clip-on, clip-off system; and post and nut.

Orangewood stick (17)–you can never have too many of these since they are used in almost every type of nail art and in nail care routines. They are inexpensive and can be purchased in bulk packs.

Sable glitter dust brush–designed for use with glitter dust powder and liquid mixer.

Stencils–no different from the stencils used by children or when home-decorating, only very much smaller. A sheet may contain stencils linked by a common theme (flowers, for example) or a selection of shapes, patterns, and popular images. You can make your own stencils with "Frisket" film or masking tape.

Stick-ons (19)–self-adhesive lines, stripes, repeat patterns, glitter patterns, and decorations that are positioned on dry polish or nail paint.

Stick-on nails (20)–see page 11.

If you decide to take nail art seriously, then you will find yourself with this array of equipment. Some items can be found in drugstores and pharmacies, but others can only be sourced through specialist nail art suppliers.

Striping brush–the long bristles are used to paint fine lines using the side of the brush.

The perfect manicure

No matter whether you decide to go wild with a nail art design or opt for an *au naturel* French polish design, the condition of your nails is important. A manicure will provide a smooth nail plate on which nail art can be created, but it will also ensure that your nails remain in top condition while wearing nail polish or nail extensions. And because your nails will be attracting a lot of deserved attention, your hands need to be beautiful–massaged to improve circulation and moisturized to undo the daily ravages of exposure to detergents.

A home manicure should be done weekly; a hand massage and moisturizing daily. Try to have a salon manicure about every couple of months. This ten-step manicure takes about 15 to 30 minutes, and the hand massage ten minutes.

You will need:

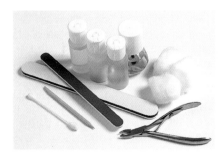

- salt
- almond or olive oil
- acetone-free nail polish remover
- cotton wool
- emery board
- orangewood stick
- bowl and warm water
- cuticle removing cream
- cuticle nippers
- moisturizing hand cream
- nail buffer
- base coat

STEP 1
Exfoliate–remove dead skin cells–by rubbing your hands and nails with salt mixed with a few

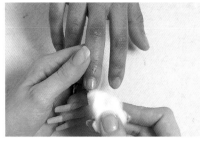

drops almond or olive oil. Lightly soak a piece of cotton wool with polish remover and wipe it over each nail to remove polish.

STEP 2
Use the finest-grain emery board to file and shape your nails. Hold the file at an angle to the nail, and file in one direction with a sweeping not a back-and-forth

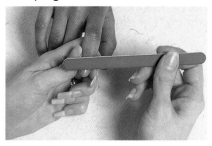

sawing movement. Work from the sides to the middle of the nail tip. Aim for a nail tip shape that is slightly square, and do not file deeply into the sides.

STEP 3
Soak the fingers of one hand in warm water, to which softening rosewater can be added, for five minutes. Then, use an orangewood stick, the tip wrapped in cotton wool, to clean behind the nails. Apply a cuticle remover or rub in oil.

STEP 4
Gently push back the cuticles–rough treatment causes dents or ridges in the nail–with an

orangewood stick. If you have not done a manicure recently, the cuticles may need to be trimmed with cuticle nippers. Do this gently and do not cut the cuticle too low. Nail technicians use cuticle nippers sparingly, so try to follow their sound practice. Refill the bowl with warm water and repeat steps 3 and 4 with the other hand.

STEP 5
Rub in a hand and nail moisturizing cream until it has all been absorbed. Now would be a good time to enjoy a hand massage (see opposite).

STEP 6
Give nails a natural glow and improve circulation by buffing, with or without a buffing paste. Buff each nail for no longer than a few seconds.

STEP 7
Wipe each nail with an acetone-free nail polish remover or an astringent such as lemon juice or witch hazel. This will remove any oil or grease from the nail plate that will interfere with the polishing process.

STEP 8
Apply a base coat, starting from the cuticle end of the nail and use just one, smooth stroke to reach the nail tip. You should be able to cover the nail in two or three

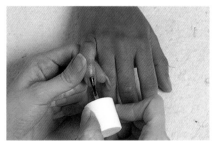

strokes. Some nail technicians recommend painting base coat behind the nail tip. At this stage, extensions and stick-on nails can be applied, or you apply polish.

Hand massage

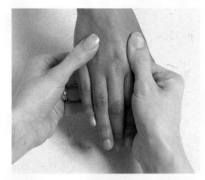

STEP 1
Remove all jewelry, then apply a generous dollop of hand massage cream (or oil) onto the palm of one hand. Spread it to cover the whole hand from fingertips to wrist.

STEP 2
Using the thumb and forefinger of the other hand, gently then firmly stroke from the fingertips to the wrist of the hand being massaged. Work from the little finger to the thumb, covering all sides. Repeat the process to massage the other hand.

STEP 3
Apply more cream or oil, but this time massage from wrist to fingertips using the same technique. Repeat steps 1-3 for the other hand.

STEP 4
To get the maximum relaxation effect, swathe your hands in a soft towel and lay them on your lap for a couple of minutes. Close your eyes and relax.

Your feet deserve to be treated to lavish care and attention. But don't stop at a pedicure and polish, let your imagination loose and create some toe-tapping nail art designs.

Treat your feet

Often the most neglected parts of our body are our feet. A sad state considering that in ancient Egypt kissing the feet was a gesture equal to a Renaissance kiss on the hand. This injustice can be corrected by regularly carrying out this 20-minute pedicure routine.

STEP 1
Remove any nail polish, then trim the nails by cutting straight across. Do not cut them too short, nor down at the corners. Smooth the edges with a flexible emery board–a medium- to coarse-grade one may be needed for strong toe nails–working from the sides to the middle in one direction.

STEP 2
Soak your feet for five minutes in warm water to which rosewater, lavender oil, or almond oil can be added. Exfoliate with a pumice stone or nail brush. Dry feet thoroughly, especially between the toes.

STEP 3
While the cuticles are still soft, push them back gently with an orangewood stick or a cotton bud dipped in oil, or apply a cuticle remover and follow the instructions on the container. Trim the cuticles with cuticle nippers only as a last resort. Buff the nail plates.

STEP 4
Wipe over the nails with acetone-free nail polish remover to remove any oil or grease, before applying a base coat and polish. Apply polish to toes by painting a semi-circle of polish at the cuticle end. Paint the middle of the nail from cuticle to tip, and use as few strokes as possible to paint the sides. Try to run the brush over the nail tip to provide extra protection.

When dry, treat your feet to a moisturizing cream or an invigorating peppermint-, rosemary- or lavender-based lotion or oil.

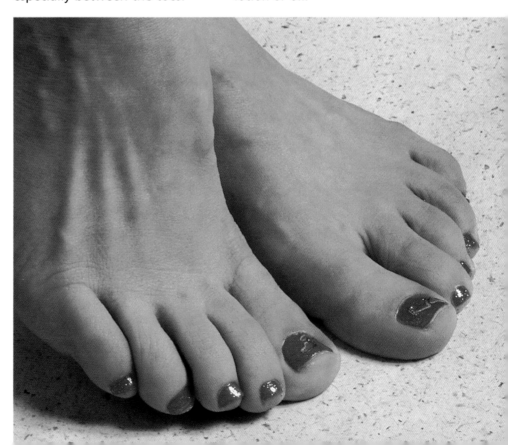

Farewell to art

The care and patience needed when manicuring and creating nail art must also be exercised when removing polish, nail art acrylics, paint, decorations, jewelry, and nail extensions. Remember, your nails are a canvas for future creations and must be treated accordingly. Rough or abrasive treatment could mean leaving your nails undecorated for a long period of time so they regain strength and condition.

Removing nail art

Remove any ring, clip-on or post jewelry. Wash, then dry it thoroughly or leave on sunny sill. If you are not going to be wearing your nail jewelry, wrap it in tissue and store safely.

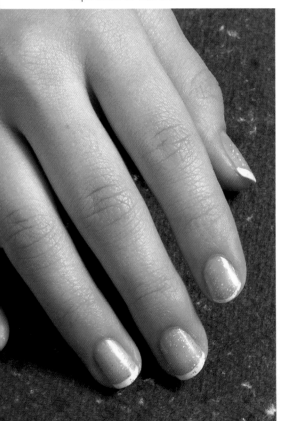

A beautiful French polish design–the most elegant and understated expression of nail art.

The most important element is to buy and use a good polish remover. A poor quality one is often little better than household paint stripper. It will dry your nails and remove the micro-organisms that are present on healthy nails. What you want is an acetone-free polish remover. Spend time reading the ingredients label on the bottles to get exactly the right product.

Removing multiple layers of polish and top coats, stick-ons and transfers can make this a 15-minute, not a two-minute task, so make sure you give yourself plenty of time.

First, saturate a ball or pad of cotton wool with remover and lay it onto the nail for a second or two to soften the polish. Then, firmly drag the cotton wool down the nail, from cuticle to nail tip. Do not use a rubbing movement. Rubbing doesn't speed up the process, it contributes to drying the skin around your nails, and streaks nail color onto your fingers. Renew the cotton ball or pad as often as necessary.

Use the tip of an orangewood stick, a pair of tweezers, or "Taper-point" tool to gently lift off loosened polish-secure, self-adhesive, and glued-on decorations. Put aside those decorations that can be used again. Don't try to force off a decoration, simply apply more polish remover to the area.

To clean polish from around the cuticle area, sides, and behind the nail tip (this area may also have been painted with a base coat, nail hardener, or top coat), use a cotton bud or orangewood stick wrapped with cotton wool and dipped in remover. As before, lay the soaked cotton ball onto the

area for a second before using a gentle stroke to remove the polish. Don't scrub or roughly push the orangewood stick under the cuticle or nail tip.

Wash your hands with a mild soap in warm water, dry thoroughly, and then go on to do a manicure (see page 14-15) or rub nurturing oil around and over the nails, and treat your hands to some intensive moisturizing. It is not enough to do this once, you must get into a regular routine of hand and nail care.

Removing stick-on nails

Put a drop of glue solvent into the sides of the nail plate and place fingertips in warm water. Once the glue has softened, the nails can be peeled off. Clean the nail plate with glue solvent to remove any stubborn glue, then wash your hands thoroughly. Go on to manicure and moisturize your nails.

Removing nail extensions

This process varies according to the sort of extensions you have. Acrylic extensions, for example, are removed by patiently soaking the fingertips in acetone and waiting for the acrylic and the tip to dissolve. You may have to resort to a little gentle persuasion with the tip of an orangewood stick to prise away stubborn remains. The crucial thing is not to damage the nail plate by accidentally removing a layer of nail along with the extension. Whenever acetone is used, follow-up with an intensive moisturizing regime.

1

Polish-secure Designs

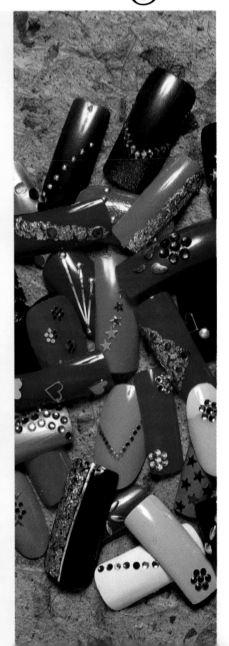

This is the easiest and quickest method of decorating one or all of your nails. All you have to do is place decorations onto your nail while the nail polish is still wet. The nail polish acts just like an adhesive, holding rhinestones, flatstones, "Dazzells", foil leaf, charms, studs, and pearls in position.

To pick up and position tiny decorations, moisten the end of an orangewood stick or blunt cocktail stick by dabbing it on a wet sponge. Alternatively, lightly dab the end of the orangewood stick with clear nail polish. The latter method has to be executed quickly or the decoration will stick fast to the orangewood stick. Larger decorations, like goo-goo eyes and charms, can be handled with tweezers. Arrange the decorations on a clean, non-greasy sheet of paper or in a shallow container, flat-side down. It is the flat surface that is lightly pressed into the wet nail polish. If the nail polish dries before you complete your design, apply a coat of clear nail polish to the nail, continue your nail art and finish with another coat of clear polish. Because polish-secure designs cover only a small part of each

nail, it is important that the nail polish is applied smoothly and evenly. As a matter of habit, always apply a base coat, two coats of a quality nail polish, and finish with a clear nail polish or strengthening and protecting top coat.

Some polish-secure items that are made of a sequin-type material will leave streaks of color across your nail if brushed over with clear nail polish or top coat. Avoid this by placing a large blob of the polish at the cuticle end of the nail and then "roll" it gently under the brush to cover the nail and the decoration. The aim is to make sure that the brush never actually touches the decoration.

Many polish-secured decorations can be used again, so take care when removing them (see page 16). They can be cleaned with nail polish remover.

Rhinestone flower

A very simple, but very effective design on colored or clear polish. You can position the flower anywhere on the nail, making sure that there is enough space around the center rhinestone to position the "petal" rhinestones. The center rhinestone can be a different color to the others. Depending on the color of the nail polish and rhinestones, this design can be dainty and subtle, or vibrant and striking.

You will need:

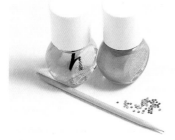

- base coat
- blue frosted nail polish
- 7 tiny blue rhinestones per nail
- orangewood stick
- clear nail polish

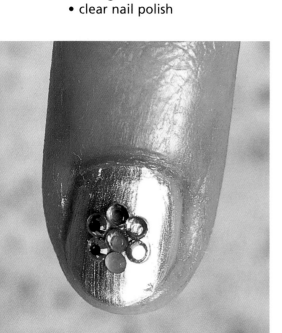

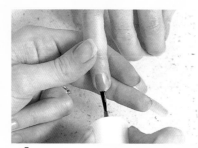

1 Apply a base coat and one coat of blue nail polish to all nails and allow to dry thoroughly.

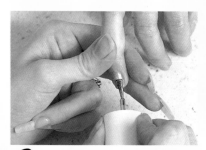

2 Working on one nail at a time, apply a second coat of blue nail polish.

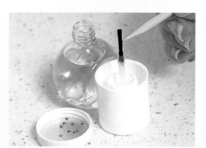

3 Dampen with water or dab with clear nail polish, the orangewood stick and pick up a rhinestone.

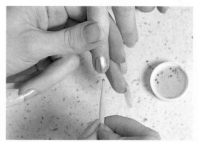

4 Working quickly, position the rhinestone–flat-side down–to make the center of the flower.

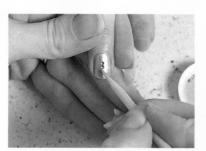

5 Position one rhinestone above and one below the center rhinestone. Try to keep the spacing even.

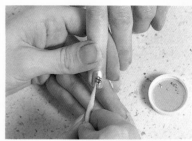

6 Add rhinestones to the right and to the left of the center one. Finish with a coat of clear nail polish.

Clowning around

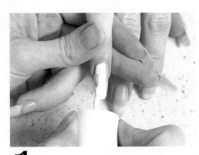

1 Apply a base coat and one coat of white nail polish to all nails. Allow to dry. Apply a second coat of white polish to the nail to be decorated.

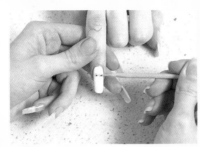

2 Working quickly while the polish is still wet, position the goo-goo eyes one-third of the way down the nail.

A cheeky, fun design that will bring a smile to everyone's face. The smiling clown-face is a particular favorite with young children and teenagers.

You will need:

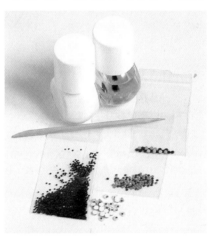

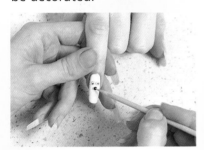

3 Position the medium-size black rhinestone centered below the eyes for the nose.

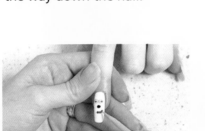

4 Position a red rhinestone centered below the nose. Add more rhinestones left and right to form the mouth.

- base coat
- white nail polish
- orangewood stick
- 2 small goo-goo eyes, 1 medium-size black rhinestone 5 tiny red rhinestones, and 6 black flatstones per nail.
- clear nail polish

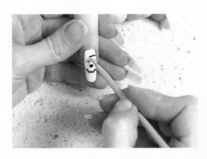

5 Starting from the center and working outward, position the black flatstones to form the eyebrows. Finish with clear nail polish, taking care that the brush does not make contact with the flatstones (see page 17).

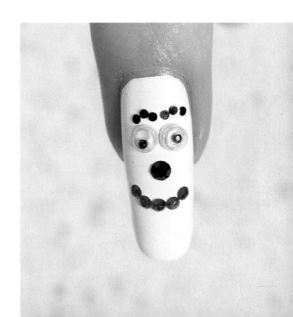

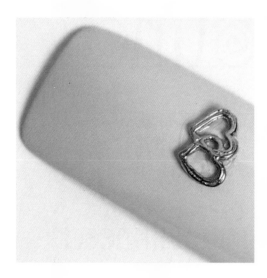

Simply charming

1. Apply a base coat and one coat of nail polish to all nails, and allow to dry. Apply a second coat of polish to the nail to be decorated.

2. Pick up the charm with the tweezers and press it into the wet polish. The charm should lay smoothly on the nail.

3. When the pink nail polish is dry, finish with a coat of clear nail polish.

You will need: base coat, pale pink nail polish, 1 charm per nail, a pair of tweezers, and clear nail polish.

Stud work

1. Apply a base coat and one coat of gloss nail polish to all nails, and allow to dry.

2. Apply a second coat of polish to the nail to be decorated. Working quickly, use a dampened orangewood stick to pick up and position the tiny studs. Start near the cuticle.

3. As you near the nail tip, start to use the small studs. Finish with a coat of clear nail polish.

You will need: base coat, dark gloss nail polish, tiny and small gold (or silver) studs, orangewood stick, and clear nail polish.

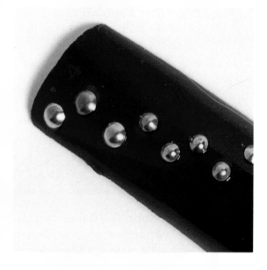

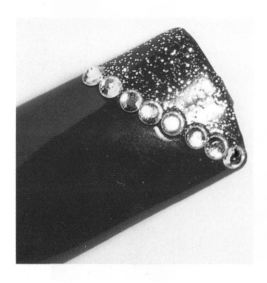

Sparkling diamonds

1. Apply a base coat and one coat of nail polish to all nails. Allow to dry. Apply a second coat of polish to the nail to be decorated.

2. While wet, position the diamonds in a diagonal line running from one corner of the nail tip to a side edge.

3. Paint the nail tips with silver sparkle nail polish. When dry, finish with clear nail polish.

You will need: base coat, red nail polish, about 8 diamond crystals per nail, orangewood stick, silver sparkle nail polish, and clear nail polish.

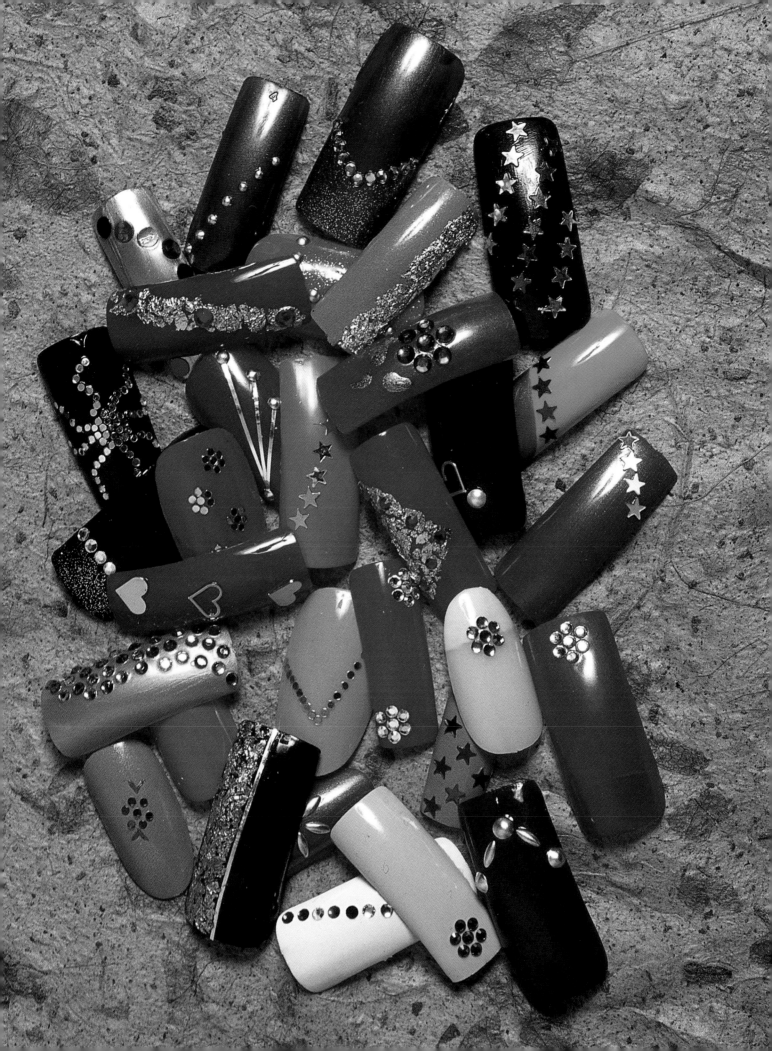

Foil leafing

There are many wonderful effects that can be achieved with gold or silver nail foil. The one shown here uses crushed foil pieces to create a striking sweep of silver across one or all nails. Vary this design by using a mixture of silver and gold foil.

You will need:

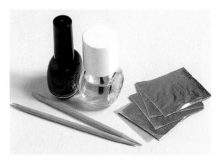

- base coat
- dark blue nail polish
- sheet of silver nail foil
- two orangewood sticks and a pair of tweezers (optional)
- clear nail polish

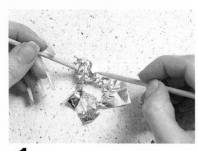

1 Use the points of the sticks to tear off tiny pieces of foil. You will need 5-7 pieces for each nail.

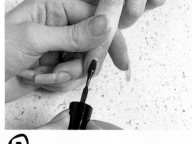

2 Apply a base coat and one coat of nail polish to all nails. Allow to dry. Apply a second coat of polish to the nail to be decorated.

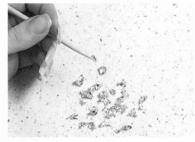

3 Pick up each piece of foil using a dampened orangewood stick or pair of tweezers.

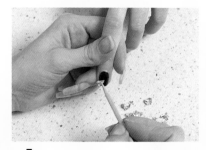

4 Position a piece of foil in a corner of the nail tip. Press the foil onto the polish, keeping the crushed-look.

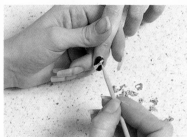

5 Work quickly to form a line of foil pieces diagonally across the nail. Finish with a coat of clear nail polish.

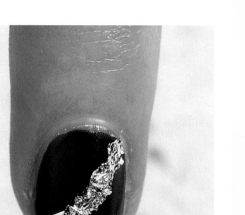

Flatstones

1. Apply a base coat and one coat of nail polish to all nails. When dry, apply a second coat of polish to the nail to be decorated.

2. Starting from the center of the nail tip, position flatstones in straight line. Try to keep the spacing even.

3. When dry, apply a coat of silver sparkle nail polish, making sure the polish brush does not touch the flatstones.

You will need: base coat, lilac nail polish, tiny purple flatstones, orangewood stick, and silver sparkle nail polish.

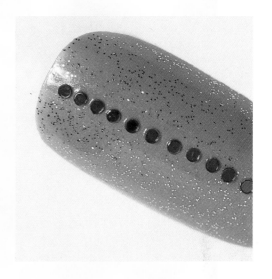

Pearl drops

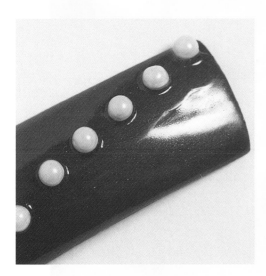

1. Apply a base coat and one coat of nail polish to all nails. When dry, apply a second coat of polish to the nail to be decorated.

2. Position one pearl in a corner of the nail tip, another near the cuticle in the opposite corner.

3. Apply pearls, evenly-spaced, to form a diagonal line. Finish with a coat of clear nail polish.

You will need: base coat, crimson nail polish, about 8 pearls per nail, orangewood stick, and clear nail polish.

Be-dazzled!

1. Apply a base coat and one coat of nail polish to all nails. When dry, apply a second coat of polish to the nail to be decorated.

2. Working quickly, position the stars to form a line down one side of the nail. Try to keep the spacing equal.

3. Finish with a coat of clear nail polish.

You will need: base coat, pale pink nail polish, star-shaped "Dazzells", orangewood stick, and clear nail polish.

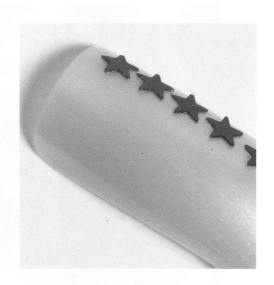

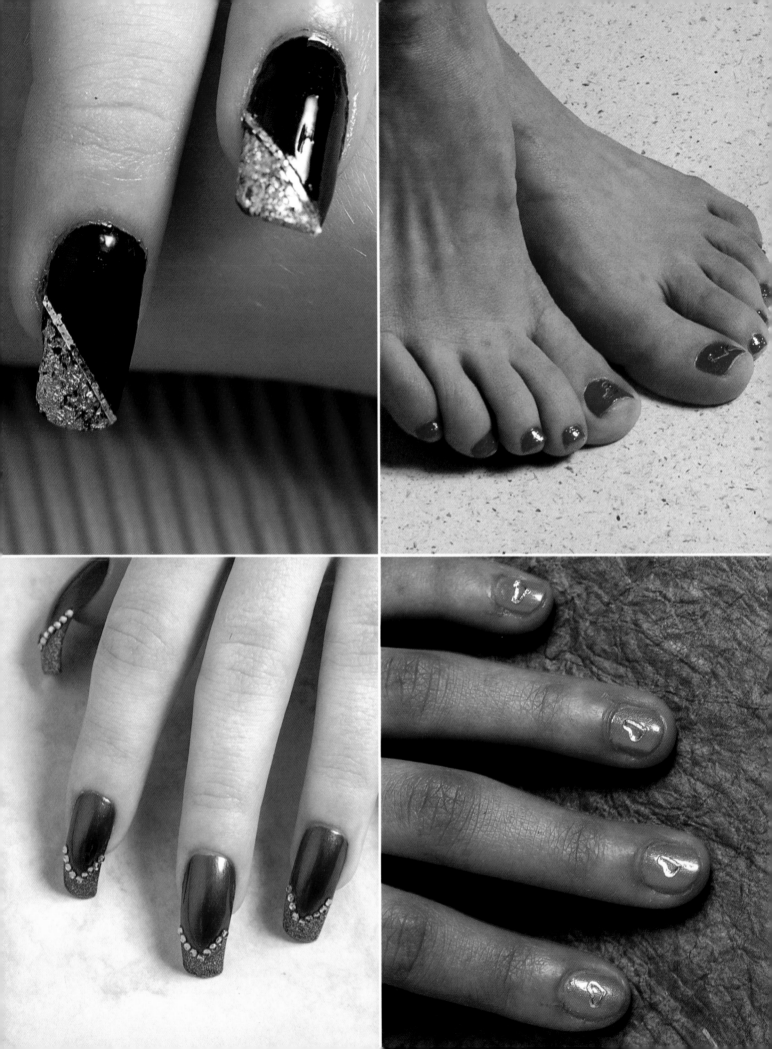

Stick-on Art

2

This form of nail art uses decorations that have a self-adhesive surface. Stick-on decorations are only ever applied to dry nail polish. Individual designs come on shiny backing paper and are easily removed with a pair of tweezers. All you have to do is position the design on your nail. Once on the nail, rolls or strips of repeat patterns or stripes need to be trimmed using a small pair of sharp-pointed, straight scissors.

Strips of repeat patterns–for example, hearts, dots and squares–come on lengths of clear adhesive, similar to sticky tape. When you have positioned the adhesive strip on your nail, obscure its edges by smoothing over with a cotton bud or orangewood stick. Trim striping tape a fraction below the nail tip to prevent the end lifting. Most nail technicians would also fix the ends of the striping tape with a drop of nail glue.

Protect stick-on nail art with two coats of clear nail polish or top coat. Apply a further protective coat of clear polish every couple of days.

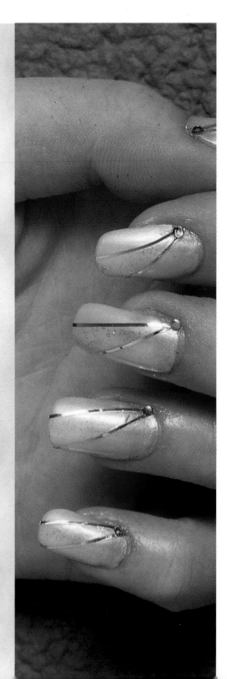

Stripes on parade

Striping tapes are available in plain, multi-colored, glitter, and metallic finishes, and also in snakeskin. While striping tapes give you perfect lines that would be impossible using a brush, you may need help positioning the tape on your nails.

You will need:

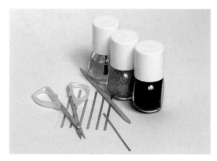

- base coat
- black nail polish
- narrow, textured gold striping tape
- scissors
- cotton bud or orangewood stick
- clear sparkle nail polish
- clear nail polish

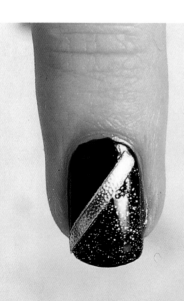

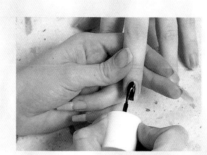

1 Apply a base coat and two coats of nail polish to all nails.

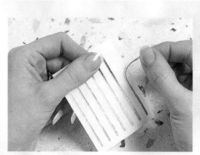

2 When nails are dry, peel a length of striping tape off the backing paper.

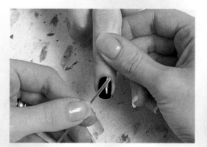

3 Position one end of the striping tape near the cuticle, angled so that it will run diagonally to the nail tip.

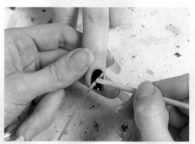

4 Smooth the striping tape, especially its edges, with a cotton bud or orangewood stick.

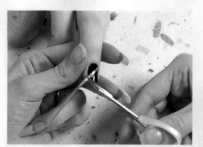

5 Trim and secure the striping tape (see page 25). Decorate other nails, making sure that the tape runs in the same direction.

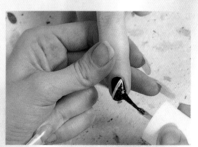

6 Apply sparkle nail polish to the tips. When dry, apply two coats of clear nail polish and further coats every few days.

Line up

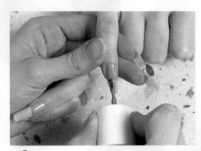

1 Apply a base coat and two coats of lilac nail polish to all nails.

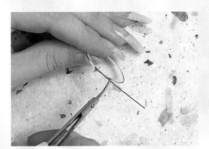

2 When nails are dry, cut a length of striping tape longer than the nail.

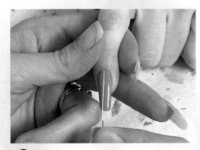

3 Position one end in the center of the nail against the cuticle. Lay the tape in a straight line to the nail tip.

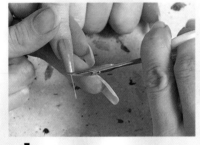

4 Smooth the tape with an orangewood stick or cotton bud. Trim the tape a fraction below the nail tip.

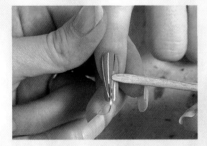

5 Follow the same routine to position angled lines either side of the center line. The lines should meet at the nail tip. Finish with two coats of clear nail polish, and do top-up coats regularly.

Use striping tape designs to flatter the shape of your nails. This pattern will make broad nails appear long and slender.

You will need:

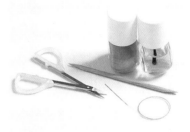

- base coat
- lilac nail polish
- roll of narrow, silver striping tape
- scissors
- cotton bud or orangewood stick
- clear nail polish

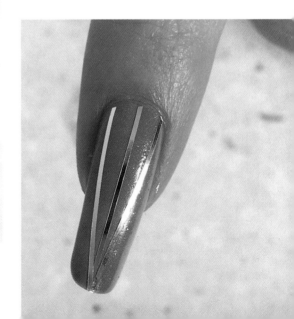

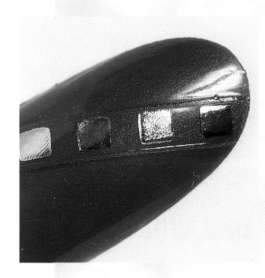

Go geometric

1. Apply a base coat and two coats of nail polish to all nails. When dry, cut a length of tape longer than the diagonal distance across the nail.

2. Remove the backing paper and position the tape on the nail. Trim so that the tape does not overhang the nail tip.

3. Smooth with a cotton bud or orangewood stick, working from the center outward. Finish with two coats of clear nail polish.

You will need: base coat, blue nail polish, square-patterned self-adhesive tape, scissors, cotton bud or orangewood stick, and clear nail polish.

Jewel finish

1. Apply a base coat and two coats of nail polish to all nails. Allow to dry thoroughly.

2. Use tweezers to lift a jewel off the backing sheet and position it near the nail tip. Depending on the length of your nails, position one or two more jewels to complete the design.

3. Press the jewels to make sure they are firmly fixed. Protect with two coats of clear nail polish, and regular top-up coats.

You will need: base coat, deep pink nail polish, sheet of stick-on jewels, pair of tweezers, and clear nail polish.

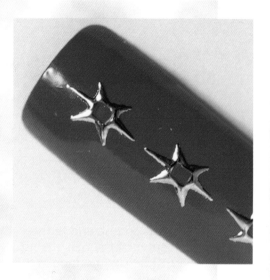

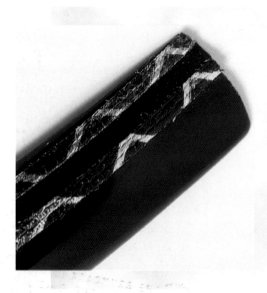

Snakeskin stripes

1. Apply a base coat and two coats of black nail polish to all nails. When dry, cut two lengths of striping tape longer than the nail.

2. Peel off the backing sheet and position one tape along the center-line of the nail. Lay the second tape parallel.

3. Smooth the tapes with a damp cotton bud or orangewood stick, and trim the ends. Finish with two coats of clear nail polish.

You will need: base coat, black nail polish, snakeskin striping tape, scissors, cotton bud or orangewood stick, and clear nail polish.

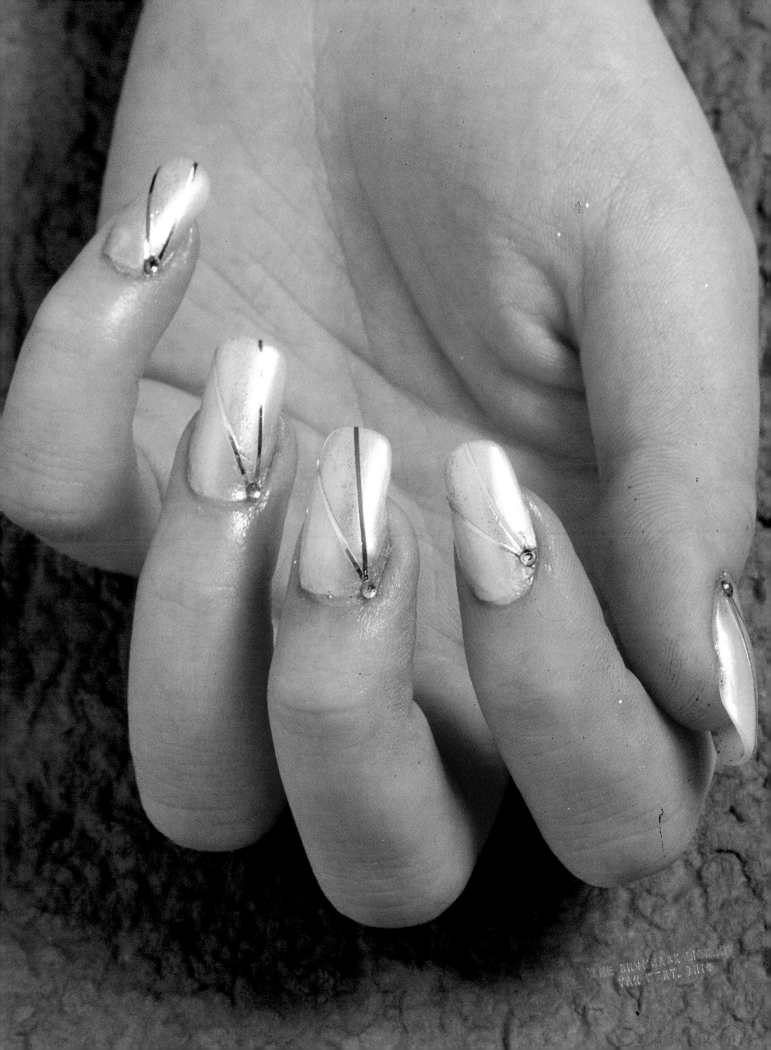

Diamond snake

The snakeskin pattern is self-adhesive, but the diamonds are polish-secured in a coat of clear nail varnish. Create your own variations on this design with striping tapes and rhinestones, pearls, or flatstones.

You will need:

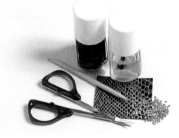

- base coat
- black nail polish
- sheet of self-adhesive silver snakeskin
- cotton bud
- 7 diamond crystals per nail
- orangewood stick
- scissors
- clear nail polish

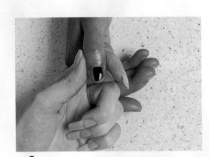

1 Apply a base coat and two coats of black nail polish to all nails, and allow to dry.

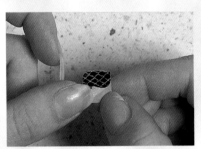

2 Cut a piece of snakeskin larger than needed and peel off the backing paper.

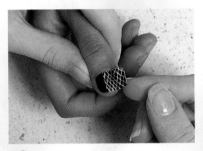

3 Position the snakeskin to cover half of the nail.

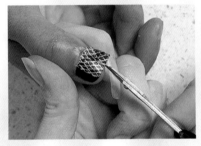

4 Smooth with a cotton bud or orangewood stick, before carefully trimming for a neat fit.

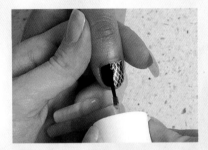

5 Apply a coat of clear nail varnish to the nail, paying attention to the join between polish and stick-on.

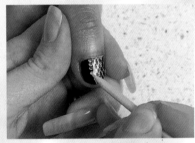

6 While wet, use a damp orangewood stick to place diamond crystals onto the polish butting the snakeskin. Finish with clear nail polish.

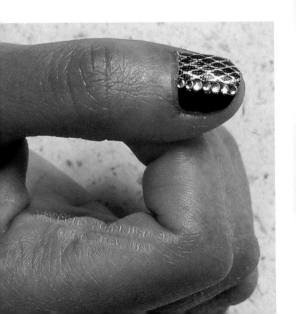

A swirl time

1. Apply a base coat and two coats of nail polish to all nails. Allow to dry. Use tweezers to peel a pattern off the backing sheet.

2. Position it in the center of the nail. Peel off two more patterns and position them above and below.

3. Smooth the patterns with a cotton bud. Protect your nail art with two coats of clear nail polish.

You will need: base coat, crimson nail polish, sheet of self-adhesive gold abstract designs, pair of tweezers, cotton bud, and clear nail polish.

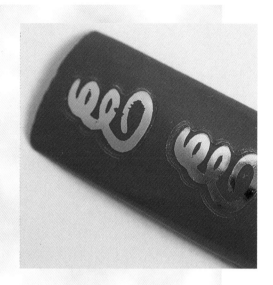

Skinned and striped

1. Apply a base coat and two coats of polish and allow to dry. Cut a piece of snakeskin larger than you will need.

2. Peel off the backing paper and position it diagonally across the upper part of the nail. Smooth and trim to fit.

3. Cut a length of striping tape longer than the nail, and position it parallel to the snakeskin. Smooth and trim. Protect your nail art with two coats of clear nail polish.

You will need: base coat, black nail polish, stick-on snakeskin, gold striping tape, scissors, cotton bud or orangewood stick, and clear nail polish.

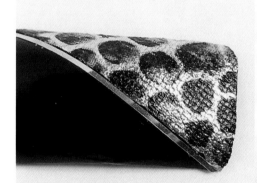

Valentine hearts

1. Apply a base coat and two coats of nail polish to all nails. Allow to dry. Use the tweezers to peel a single heart motif off the backing paper and position it near the nail tip.

2. Use the tweezers to position paired hearts in the center of the nail, and another single heart near the cuticle.

3. Smooth and seal the edges with a cotton bud or orangewood stick. Finish with two coats of clear nail polish.

You will need: base coat, pink nail polish, sheet of self-adhesive black hearts, pair of tweezers, cotton bud or orangewood stick, and clear nail polish.

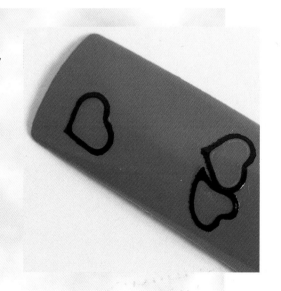

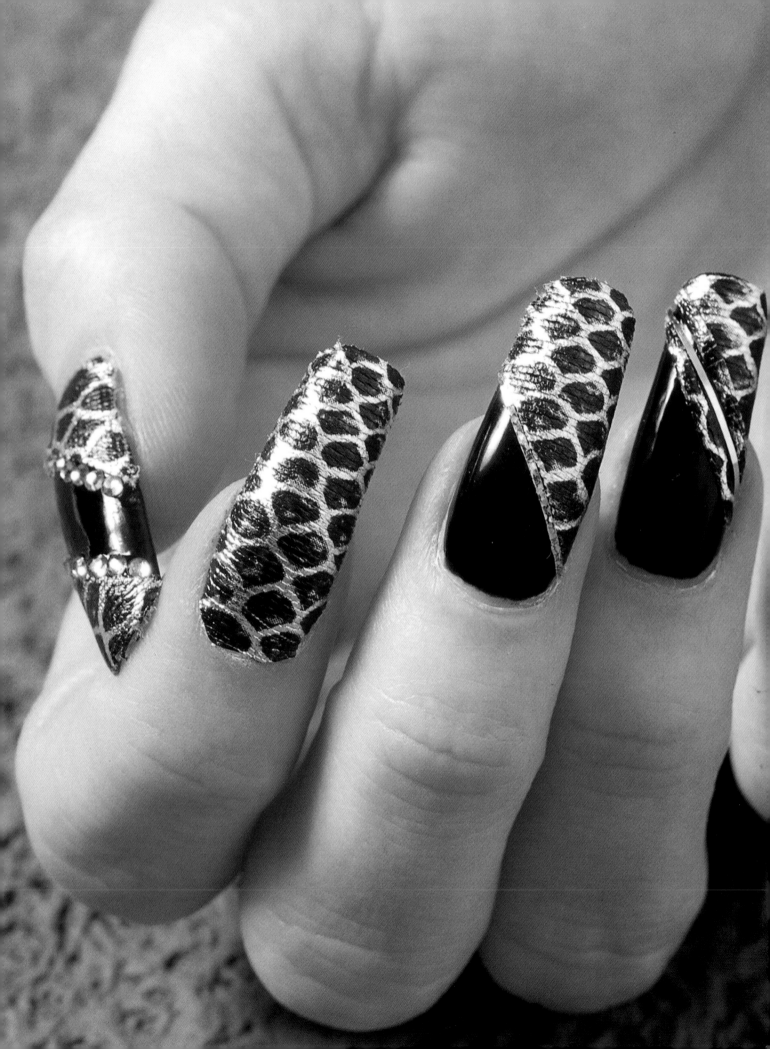

Dream Transfers

A nail art transfer is like any other transfer. A picture or pattern printed on clear film is released from its white backing sheet when dampened with water. The transfer is then placed onto dry nail polish, and once protected with clear nail polish will remain intact until removed with nail polish remover.

Transfers of different sizes come in sheets and the pictures or patterns on each sheet share a common theme. You can use just one transfer to decorate a nail, or use several in combination to create a unique design. Before settling on a design, check that the size of the transfer fits the nail on which it is to be used. Cut out the transfers needed for the nails of one hand, leaving a narrow edge around each one, and place them in the right order. Make a duplicate set of transfers for the nails of the other hand.

With your transfers cut out and your nails ready, turn over the first transfer and gently rub the backing sheet with a wet cotton bud. The color of the backing sheet will change as it absorbs the water. Wait a few moments to allow the water to fully penetrate and then, holding just the edge of the backing sheet turn over the transfer and gently slide a thumb across the design. The design will slide free of the backing paper. For small transfers, stop when you see the transparent border appear over the edge of the backing sheet and use a pair of tweezers to hold this transparent border and lift the transfer away and onto the nail. If the transfer creases or bubbles, smooth it with a damp cotton bud.

Some transfers are designed to cover the entire nail. Do not trim any excess transfer at the nail tip with scissors, but simply coat the excess with clear top coat to make it disintegrate.

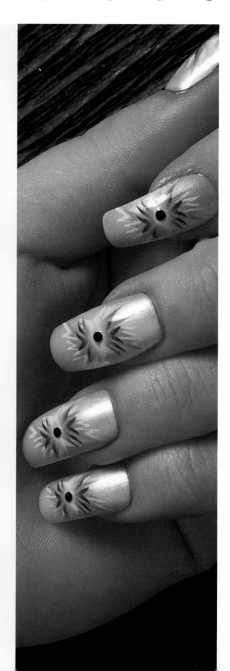

Wild thing

This gold and brown "rumble in the jungle" transfer has a wonderful embossed texture. But despite its exotic appeal, it is perfect for the work a'day routine or the all-night party. While any excess transfer at the nail tip will disappear with a coat of clear nail varnish, use scissors to trim the side edges.

You will need:

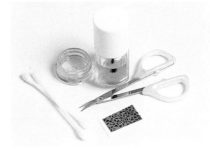

- base coat
- transfers
- scissors
- cotton buds
- container of water
- clear nail polish

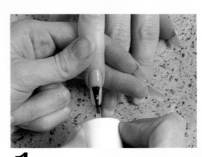

1 Apply a base coat to each nail, and allow to dry thoroughly.

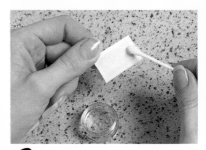

2 Dampen the backing sheet of a transfer with water. When the backing sheet changes color, turn over the transfer.

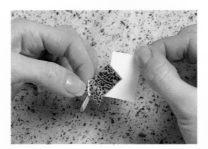

3 Hold one edge and use a thumb and forefinger to slide the transfer across and off the backing sheet.

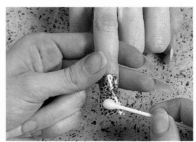

4 Position the transfer to fit neatly against the cuticle. Smooth with a damp cotton bud to remove creases.

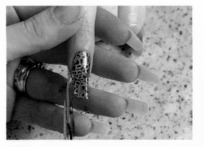

5 Use scissors to trim the side edges of the transfer to fit neatly.

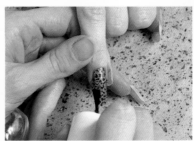

6 Apply two coats of clear nail varnish to disintegrate excess transfer at the nail tip and to protect your nail art.

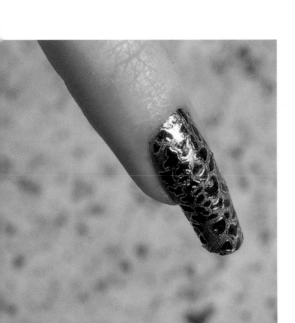

Floral bouquet

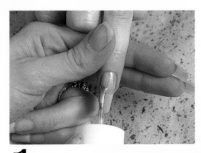

1 Varnish nails with a base coat and two coats of pale pink nail polish. Allow to dry thoroughly.

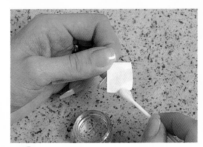

2 Use a cotton bud to dampen the backing sheet of the first transfer with water.

This transfer would have been cut from a sheet containing all sorts of variations on this floral bouquet. Some designs will best suit long nails, others will be perfect for shorter nails. It is usual, though not a rule, that a nail art design should be the right way up when viewed by someone else, but upside-down from your perspective.

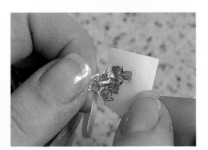

3 When the backing sheet changes color, turn over the transfer and slide the transfer free.

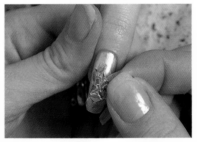

4 Use a pair of tweezers or a thumb and forefinger to place the transfer onto the nail.

You will need:

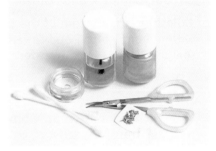

- base coat
- pale pink nail polish
- sheet of floral transfers
- scissors
- cotton buds
- container of water
- clear nail polish

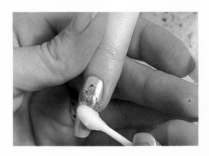

5 Smooth the transfer with a damp cotton bud, working from the center to the edges. Finish with two coats of clear nail varnish.

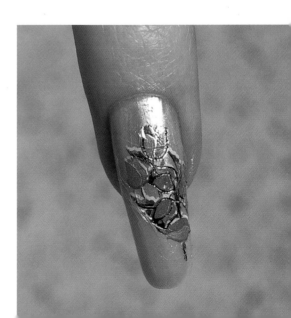

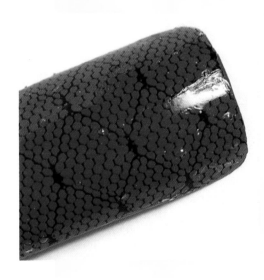

Lace netting

1. Apply a base coat and two coats of red nail polish to all nails. Allow to dry.

2. Cut out, dampen, and remove the each transfer, as shown on previous pages. Position on the nail and smooth.

3. Trim the sides with scissors, then apply two coats of clear varnish to disintegrate excess transfer and to protect the nail art.

You will need: base coat, red nail polish, wet-release black lace transfers, scissors, cotton buds, container of water, and clear nail polish.

Tropical daze

1. Apply a base coat and two coats of white nail polish to nails. Cut out, dampen, and remove the each transfer, as shown before.

2. Position the bottom of the transfer near the nail tip. Smooth with a damp cotton bud to remove creases and air bubbles and to seal the edges of the transfer.

3. Trim the sides with scissors. Apply two coats of clear nail polish to protect.

You will need: base coat, white nail polish, wet-release "tropical holiday" transfers, scissors, cotton buds, container of water, and clear nail polish.

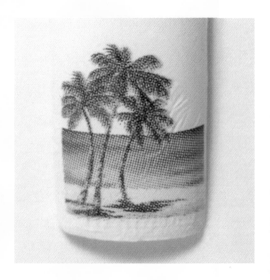

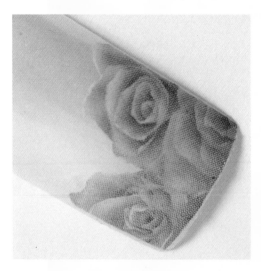

Rose tips

1. Apply a base coat and two coats of white nail polish to nails. Cut out, dampen, and remove the each transfer, as shown before.

2. Position the transfer over the nail tip. Smooth with a damp cotton bud to seal the edges of the transfer. Trim the sides and apply clear nail varnish to dissolve any overhang.

3. When dry, apply a second coat of clear nail polish.

You will need: base coat, white nail polish, wet-release floral transfers, scissors, cotton buds, container of water, and clear nail polish.

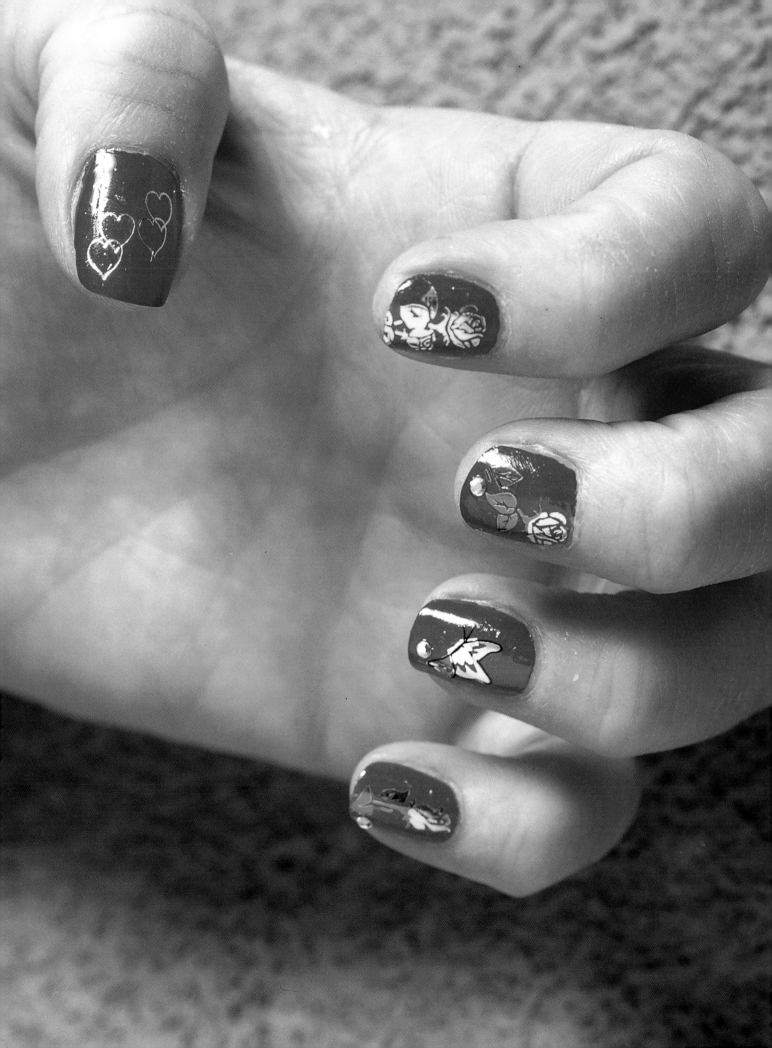

On the prowl

The image of the sleek, prowling tiger is spread over four wet-release transfers, so before starting, arrange the pieces in the correct order.

You will need:

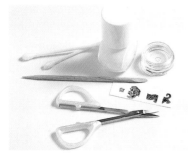

- base coat
- white nail polish
- sheet of wet-release tiger transfers
- scissors
- cotton buds
- container of water
- clear nail polish

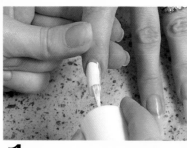

1 Apply a base coat and two coats of white nail polish to all nails.

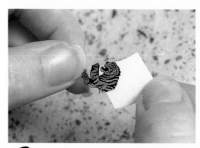

2 Dampen the back of the first transfer (the tiger's head) and remove the transfer, as shown before.

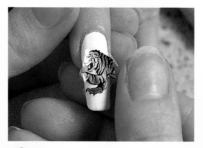

3 Position the transfer in the center of the middle finger nail.

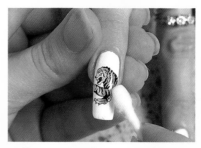

4 Smooth the transfer with a damp cotton bud to remove air bubbles and creases and to seal the edges.

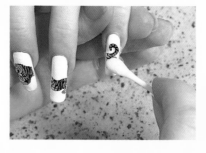

5 Follow the same steps to position the tiger's body on the ring finger, it's tail on the little finger, and front paw on the pointing finger. Finish with two coats of clear nail polish.

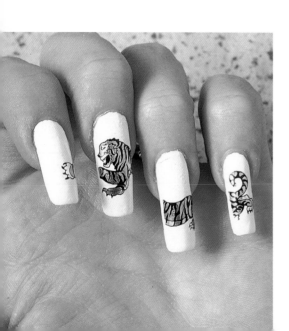

Gilded roses

1. Apply a base coat and two coats of lilac nail polish to nails. Cut out, dampen, and remove the each transfer, as shown before.

2. Position the transfer so stems are near the nail tip. Smooth with a damp cotton bud to remove creases and air bubbles and to seal the edges of the transfer.

3. Apply two coats of clear nail polish to protect and dissolve excess transfer.

You will need: base coat, lilac nail polish, metallic wet-release floral transfers, scissors, cotton buds, container of water, and clear nail polish.

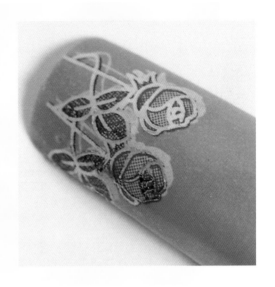

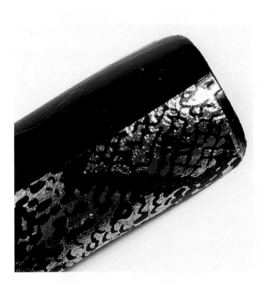

Snakes alive

1. Apply a base coat and two coats of black nail polish to nails. Cut out the snakeskin decal to cover half of each nail.

2. Dampen and remove the first decal, as shown before. Position a straight edge along the center-line of the nail.

3. Smooth with a damp cotton bud, trim sides to fit, and then apply two coats of clear nail polish.

You will need: base coat, black nail polish, wet-release snakeskin decal, scissors, cotton buds, container of water, and clear nail polish.

Arty nail

1. Apply a base coat and two coats of pink nail polish to nails. Cut out 1-3 transfers per nail. Dampen and remove the each transfer, as shown before.

2. Position the transfers to create an interesting pattern. If there is not enough room for a whole transfer, position it near the sides and trim the excess with scissors.

3. Smooth each transfer with a damp cotton bud. Finish by applying two coats of clear nail polish.

You will need: base coat, pink nail polish, metallic wet-release abstract transfers, scissors, cotton buds, container of water, and clear nail polish.

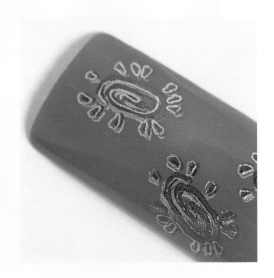

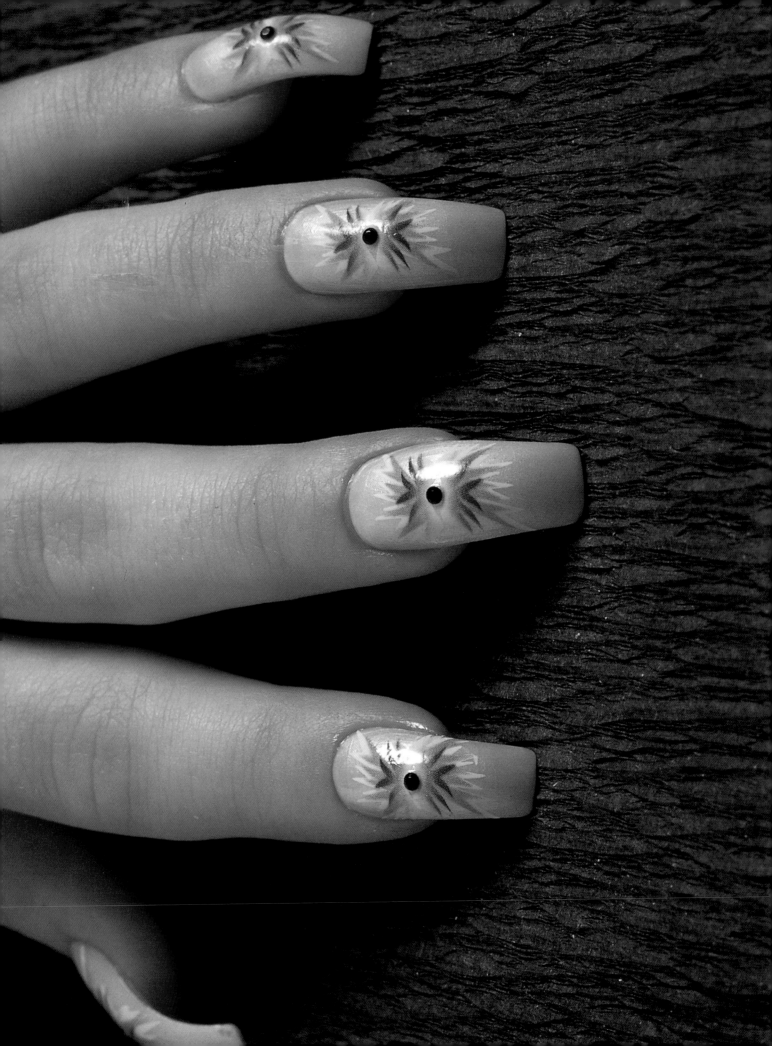

French Designs
—a polished art

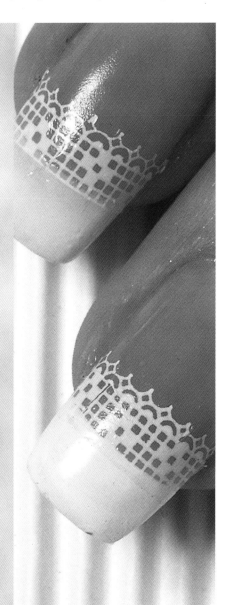

The French design, or French polish, is one of the most popular nail art creations from New York to Newcastle, Singapore to Sydney. It is a natural and clean-looking design that is suitable for all ages, and all nail shapes and lengths. It is especially attractive on short or sporty-length nails and long, square-tipped nail extensions.

The classic French polish involves painting the nail with a pale beige, pink, or cream nail polish, while the tip is varnished white or ivory. The American version of the French polish design uses a darker base color, which can often better suit dusky, dark, and sun-tanned skin tones.

The "line" separating the white tip from the base color is called the "C" curve or "smile" line. It takes practice to paint an even "C" curve, but as you will read below, clever tricks can take the place of arduous trial and error.

Where you mark the "C" curve is one of personal choice. Short nails look longer if the "C" curve is lowered toward the cuticle. Those with long nails may paint the "C" curve following the natural line on the nail.

There are several products that can help you create the perfect "C" curve, but many opt to use the cotton thread trick that you will find on page 42. Becoming increasing more popular is a guide tape. This is a specially-shaped piece of adhesive tape that you place across the nail once the base color is dry. The upper edge of the guide tape marks the "C" curve. Once the free edge is painted and dry, the guide tape is carefully removed to reveal the "C" curve.

Guide tapes are available in two forms: crescent-shaped and chevron. The crescent is the standard smile-line shape, while the chevron is "V" shaped. It is positioned so that the apex of the "V" points to the center of the nail tip.

French polish

This is the classic French polish design–pale base color, crescent "C" curve, and white tip. A simple length of cotton sewing thread will help you achieve the perfect "smile" line. Firmly tape the thread to your work surface, or knot the thread around a fixed item. Do this before applying the base color. Dampen the thread to prevent it adhering to the wet polish.

You will need:

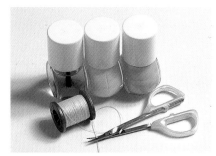

- base coat
- pale-color nail polish for the base color
- cotton sewing thread
- white nail polish for free edge
- clear nail polish

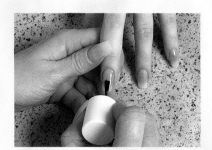

1 Apply a base coat and two coats of pale base color polish to nails.

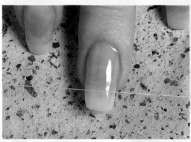

2 While the base color is tacky, slide each nail under the taut thread. Bring the thread down, guillotine-style, onto the wet polish to mark the smile line.

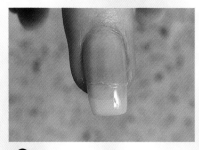

3 Quickly lift off the thread to reveal a shallow "channel" in the base color.

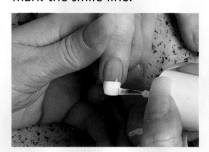

4 Apply two coats of white nail polish to the free edge, using the "channel" as a painting guide.

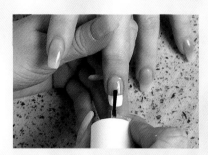

5 When dry, protect the French polish with clear nail polish. Apply a further coat every three days.

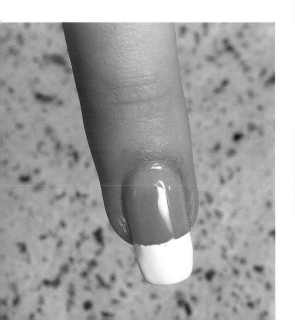

American chevron

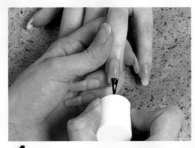

1 Apply base coat to nails.

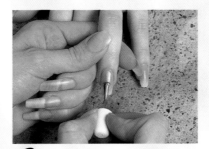

2 Follow with two coats of base-color nail polish. Allow to dry thoroughly.

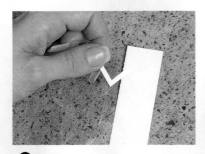

3 Working on one hand at a time, peel the chevron guide tapes off their backing sheet.

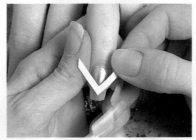

4 Position the guide tape so that upper edge marks the "V" line and the "V" points to the nail tip. Smooth the guide tapes with an orangewood stick.

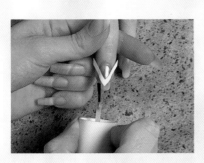

5 Paint the tip with cream nail polish. When dry, carefully peel off the guide tapes. Apply clear nail polish.

Guide tapes have made it even easier to paint a perfect "smile" line. This design shows the "V" shaped chevron guide tape, but the same method is used for a crescent-shaped guide tape.

You will need:

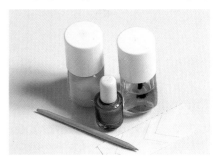

- base coat
- beige nail polish for the base color
- self-adhesive chevron guide tapes
- orangewood stick
- cream nail polish for free edge
- clear nail polish

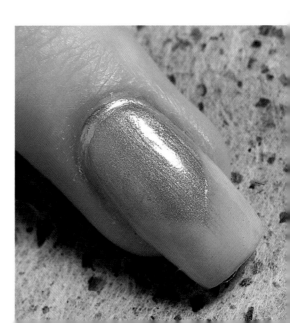

French chevron

1. Apply a base coat and two coats of a pale base-color to nails. Allow to dry thoroughly.

2. Working on one hand at a time, position the guide tapes so the upper edge marks where you want the "V" line to be. Paint the tip with two coats of white nail polish.

3. When dry, carefully peel off the guide tapes. Finish with a coat of clear nail polish.

You will need: base coat, pale nail polish for base color, chevron guide tapes, orangewood stick, white nail polish for free edge, and clear nail polish.

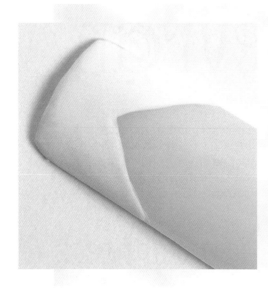

Chevron of pearls

1. Give your nails a French chevron polish following steps 1 to 5 (excluding the application of clear nail varnish) on page 43.

2. Working on one nail at a time, apply a coat of clear nail varnish and while wet, use a dampened orangewood stick to pick up and position pearls–flat-side down–along the "V" line.

3. Finish with a second coat of clear nail polish to further secure the pearls and protect the nail art.

You will need: base coat, pale nail polish for base color, chevron guide tapes, orangewood stick, white nail polish for free edge, 6-8 pearls, and clear nail polish.

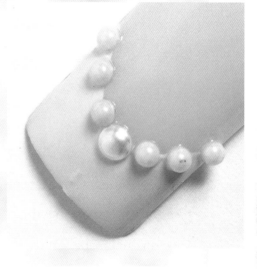

French transfer

1. Apply a base coat and two coats of black nail polish to nails, and allow to dry thoroughly.

2. Cut out, dampen, and release the transfers as shown on pages 33-39. Position each transfer along the nail tip, and smooth with a damp cotton bud to release air bubbles and creases.

3. Apply two coats of clear nail polish to protect the transfer.

You will need: base coat, black nail polish, floral chevron transfers, scissors, cotton bud, container of water, and clear nail polish.

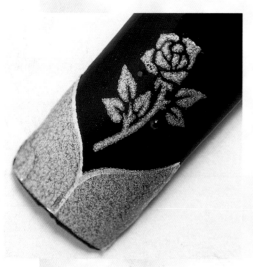

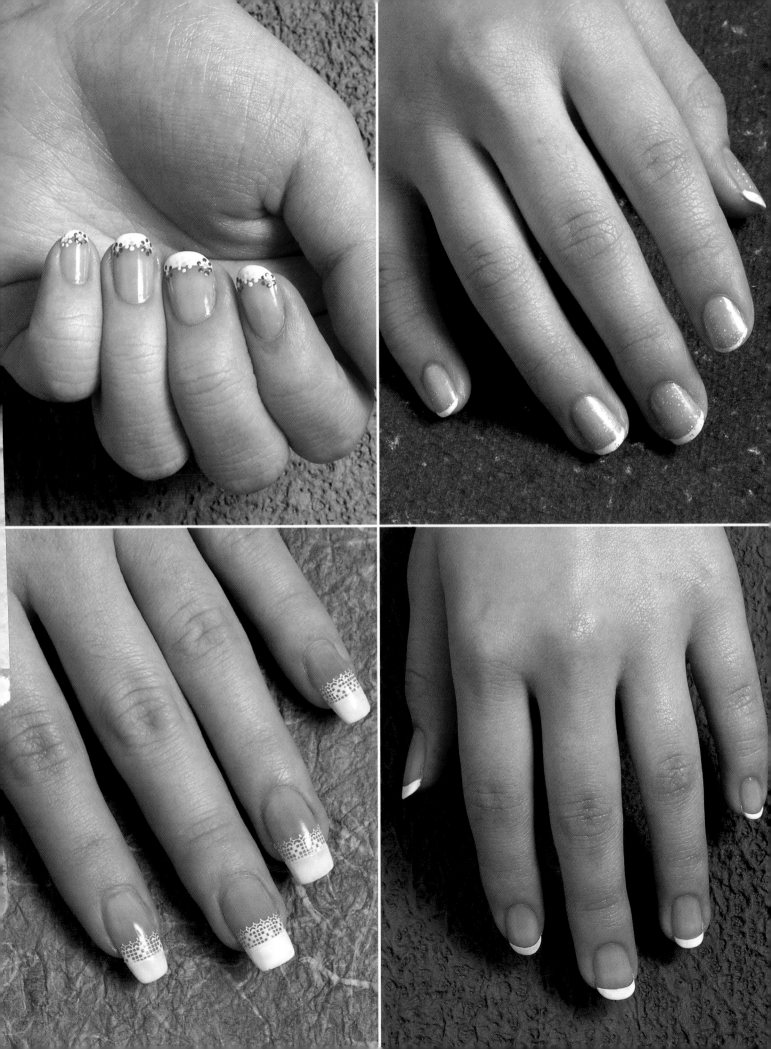

A touch of lace

There is a hint of something very "ooh-la-la" about this quietly naughty decal. The lace decal is applied once a French polish design is complete and dry, but before painting on clear nail polish. The lace decal is a sneaky way of hiding a less-than-perfect "C" curve.

You will need:

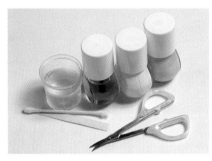

- base coat
- pale or clear nail polish for base color
- white nail polish for free edge
- sheet of wet-release, white lace decals
- scissors
- cotton bud
- container of water
- clear nail polish

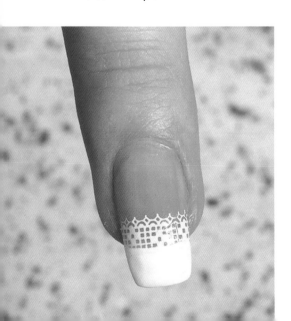

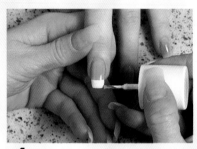

1 Apply a base coat and two coats of base color to nails. Allow to dry. Create the "C" curves and paint the free edges white.

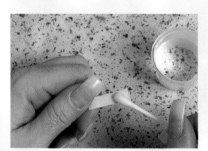

2 Cut out ten strips of lace decal longer than the width of the nails. Working on one nail at a time, use a damp cotton bud to wet the back of the decal.

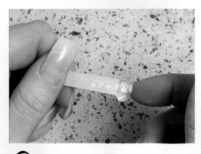

3 When the water has penetrated, turn over the decal and slide the decal off the backing paper.

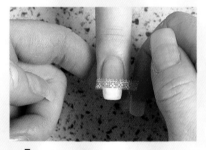

4 Using thumb and forefingers, position the decal–lacy edge furthest from nail tip–along the "C" curve.

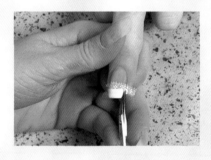

5 Smooth with a damp cotton bud, then trim the decal to fit. Finish with two coats of clear nail polish.

Glitter tipped

1. Apply a base coat and two coats of base color to nails. Allow to dry. Create the "C" curves and paint the free edge ivory.

2. Working on one nail at a time, cut a length of striping tape. Position it along the "C" curve. Smooth with the orangewood stick and trim for a neat fit.

3. Paint the free edges with sparkle nail polish. When dry, apply a coat of clear varnish.

You will need: base coat, ivory nail polish for base color, white nail polish for free edge, gold striping tape, scissors, orangewood stick, sparkle nail polish, and clear nail polish.

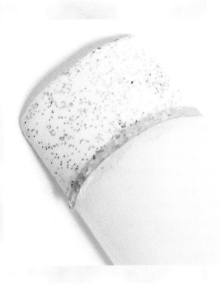

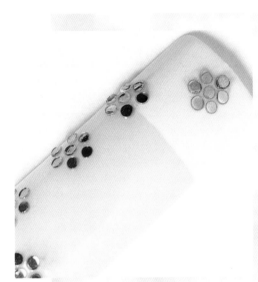

Daisy chain

1. Apply a base coat and two coats of base color to nails. Allow to dry. Create the "C" curves and paint the free edge white.

2. Working on one nail at a time, apply clear nail polish and, while still wet, use a dampened orangewood stick to position flatstones to create a daisies, starting at the nail tip.

3. Finish with a coat of clear nail polish, making sure the brush does not come in contact with the flatstones (see page 17).

You will need: base coat, ivory nail polish for base color, white nail polish for free edge, clear nail varnish, gold flatstones, and an orangewood stick.

Vive la difference!

1. Apply a base coat and two coats of while nail polish. While wet, use the cotton thread trick (see page 42) to mark the diagonal line. Paint the tip with two coats of mauve nail polish, and allow to dry.

2. Working on one nail at a time, apply a coat of clear nail polish. While wet, position the rhinestones along the diagonal line.

3. Finish with a second coat of clear nail polish.

You will need: base coat, white nail polish for base color, cotton sewing thread, mauve nail polish for tip, clear nail varnish, black rhinestones, and an orangewood stick.

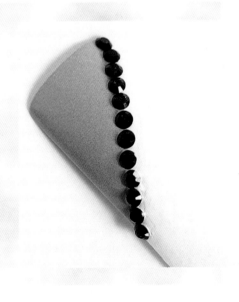

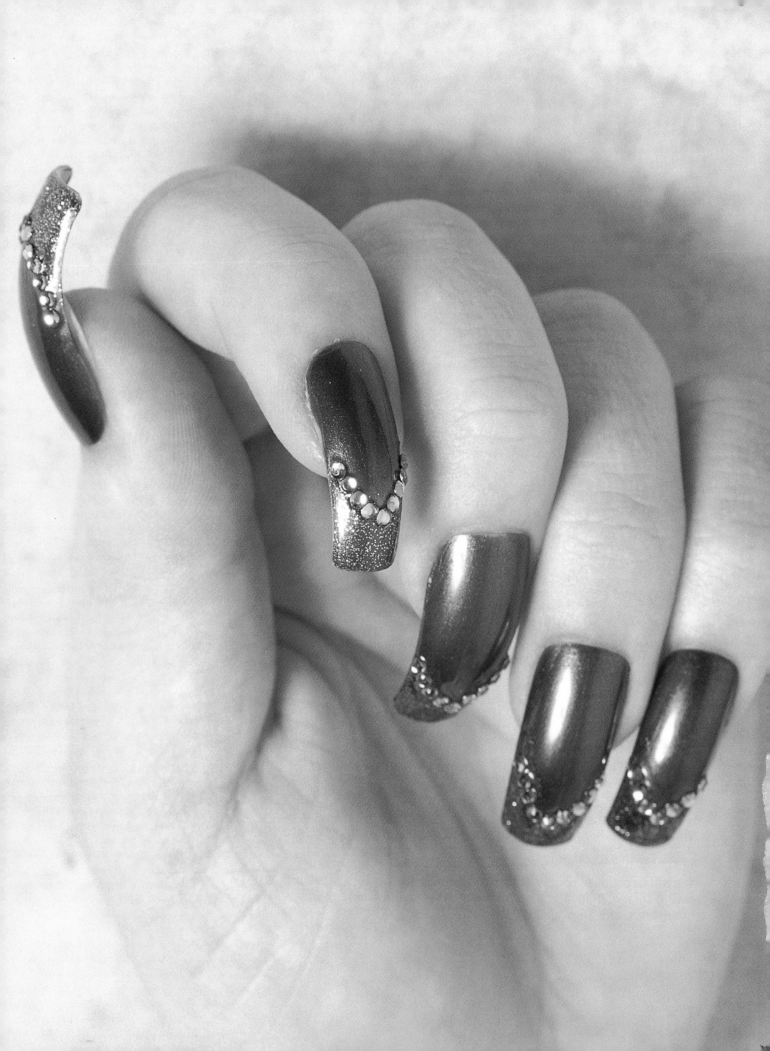

Glitter Dust 5

Glitter dust is a dry mixture of fine particles of glitter. When combined with a special mixer varnish, glitter dust forms a thick, glittery substance of a treacle-like consistency. Its consistency gives glitter dust a rich and "solid" look that sparkle nail polishes cannot equal. Glitter dust can be manipulated into different "shapes" on the nail, and it comes in about 30 colors and is available, along with the mixer varnish, from quality nail art suppliers. If you are unable to obtain the special mixer varnish, some brands of clear, thick nail polish will do the job.

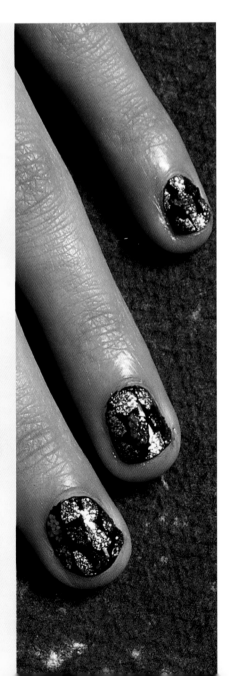

Glitter dust dries very hard and a glitter dust design will, with care, last several weeks. Because of its strength, an all-over glitter dust design will strengthen and protect weak or brittle nails.

The secret to working successfully with glitter dust is patience; work quickly and you may not mix the glitter to the best consistency. Once you've decided which colors you are going to use–for purely practical reasons limit yourself to five colors per design–dip the glitter brush into the mixer varnish. Slowly raise it a little out of the bottle and wait until you see a small ball of mixer varnish form on the tip of the brush. Gently take the brush to the pot of glitter dust and roll–not dip–the ball of mixer varnish around the surface until it is covered with glitter dust. The ball should look like a shiny bead.

Dab the ball into position on the nail. Wipe the glitter brush on a paper towel to remove excess glitter dust. Use the now-clean tip of the brush to spread the ball of glitter dust into the desired shape. Wash the glitter brush in nail polish remover before moving onto a new color and when the design is completed. Should you make a mistake or one area of glitter dust merges with another, allow to dry and then simply paint over the mistake using the base color nail polish and a fine brush.

Stained glass

Glitter dust colors and textures are deep and rich, and the resulting designs always attract admiring glances and comments. It is the perfect medium for creating a stained-glass effect.

You will need:

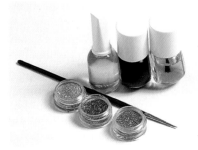

- base coat
- black nail polish
- silver, pink, and gold glitter dust
- special mixer varnish
- fine-tip glitter brush
- clear nail polish

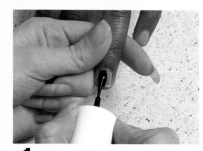

1 Apply a base coat and two coats of black nail polish to nails, and allow to dry thoroughly.

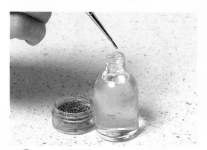

2 Dip the brush tip into mixer varnish. When the ball of mixer varnish forms at the tip, roll it on the surface of the pink glitter dust.

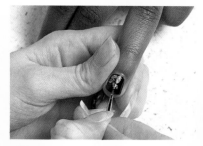

3 Dab the ball onto the nail, then wipe the brush clean. Spread the glitter dust using the brush tip. Clean the brush with polish remover before changing colors.

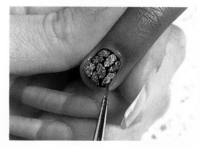

4 Leave spaces between the glitter dust so that the base color shows through.

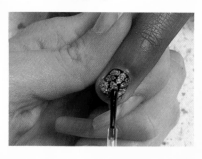

5 When the glitter dust is thoroughly dry, protect with a coat of clear nail varnish. If the glitter shapes have merged, redefine them using black acrylic paint and a fine-tip art brush.

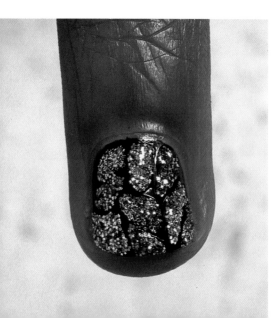

Diamonds are forever

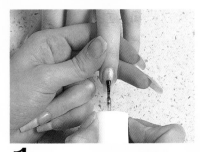

1 Apply a base coat and one coat of white nail polish. Allow to dry before applying gold sparkle nail polish.

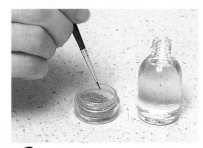

2 Dip the brush tip into mixer varnish. When a ball of mixer varnish forms on the tip, roll it on the surface of the gold glitter dust.

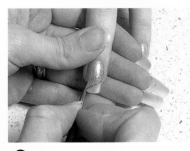

3 Dab the ball midway along one side edge. Wipe the brush clean. Drag the glitter diagonally across the nail to make a fine line. Repeat to make a parallel line.

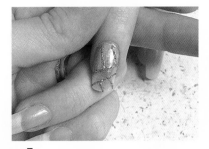

4 Follow the same method for the remaining lines. Always drag the ball of glitter dust toward the nail tip or cuticle.

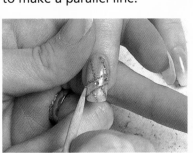

5 Working on one nail at a time, apply clear nail polish. While wet, position the diamond crystals using a dampened orangewood stick. Finish with a second coat of clear nail polish.

Glitter dust is so malleable it can be shaped or dragged to form fine lines that look like window tracery. The three diamond crystals are polish-secured into gold sparkle nail polish.

You will need:

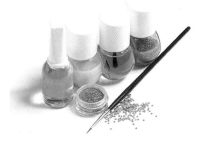

- base coat
- frosted white nail polish
- gold sparkle nail varnish
- gold glitter dust
- special mixer varnish
- fine-tip glitter brush
- 1-3 diamond crystals per nail
- orangewood stick
- clear nail polish.

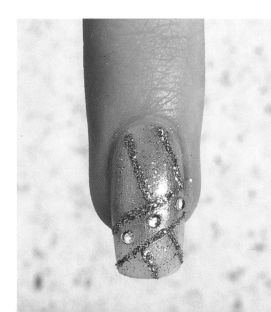

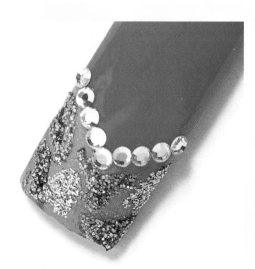

Glittering chevron

1. Follow steps 1 and 5 (excluding the application of clear polish) on page 43, using red nail polish and gold acrylic paint to create the chevron design.

2. Mix the glitter dust and apply in the usual way. Tease it to form irregular shapes. Wash the brush in polish remover before changing colors.

3. Apply clean nail varnish and position rhinestones. Finish with another coat of clear nail varnish.

You will need: base coat; red nail polish for base color; gold acrylic paint for the tip; pink, purple, and silver glitter dust; special mixer varnish; fine-tip glitter brush; clear nail polish; rhinestones; and a damp orangewood stick.

Neon shower

1. Apply a base coat and two coats of white nail polish. Allow to dry.

2. Mix the green glitter dust and apply one ball at the cuticle-end of the nail. Wipe the brush, then tease the glitter dust in to a raindrop shape.

3. Make more raindrops in green and the other colors. Clean the brush with polish remover when changing colors. When dry, apply a coat of clear nail polish.

You will need: base coat; white nail polish; green, yellow, and pink neon glitter dust; special mixer varnish; fine-tip glitter brush; and clear nail varnish.

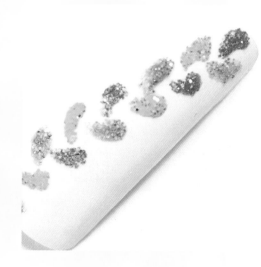

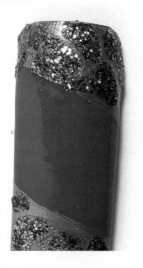

Half and half

1. Apply a base coat and two coats of red polish. Allow to dry. Paint the diagonal areas with gold acrylic paint and liner brush. Allow to dry.

2. Using the same method as used for "Glittering chevron", mix and apply balls of glitter dust and tease them to form irregular shapes on the gold-painted sections. Between each new application or color change, wipe the brush or clean with polish remover.

3. When dry, apply two coats of clear nail polish.

You will need: base coat; red nail polish for base color; gold acrylic paint; liner brush; green, gold, and purple glitter dust; special mixer varnish; fine-tip glitter brush; and clear nail polish.

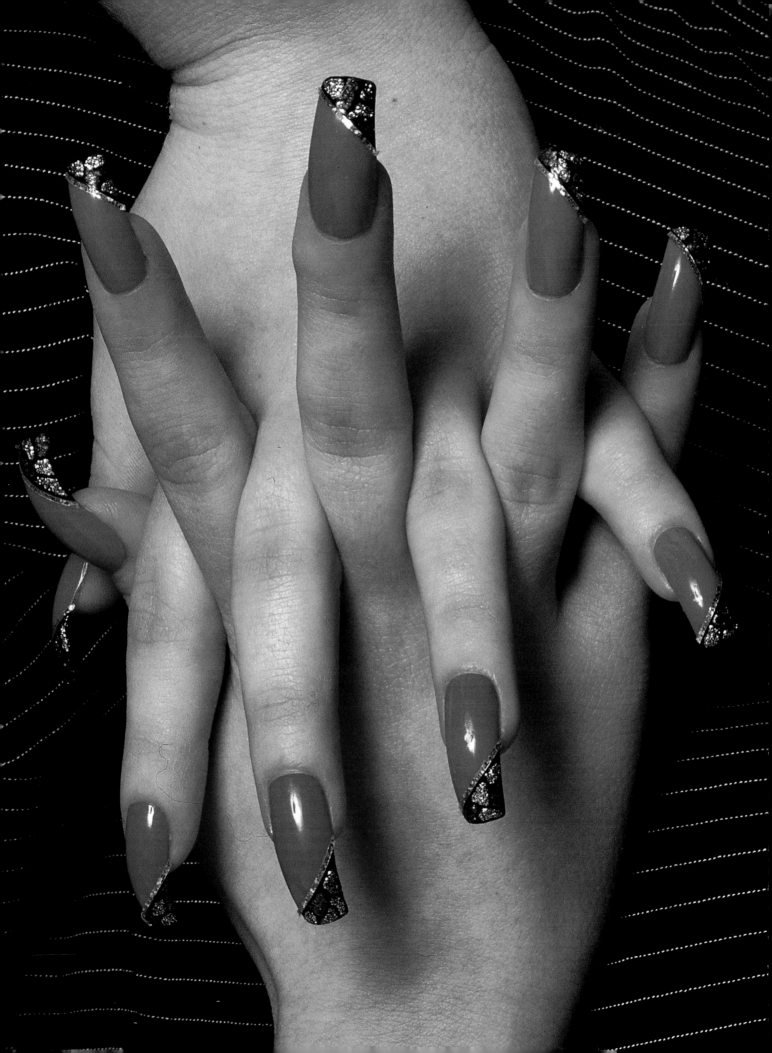

Cherries

This nail art design is easy to do with glitter dust. The glitter dust balls form perfect cherries, while the leaves need just the tiniest amount of manipulation.

You will need:

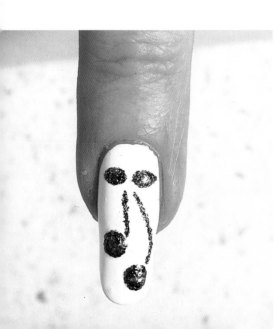

- base coat
- white nail polish
- red and green glitter dust
- special mixer varnish
- fine-tip glitter brush
- clear nail polish

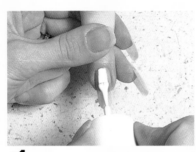

1 Apply a base coat and two coats of white nail polish and allow to dry.

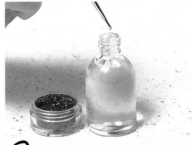

2 Dip the brush tip into the mixer varnish, and raise it out of the bottle. When the ball of mixer varnish forms, roll the ball on the surface of the red glitter dust.

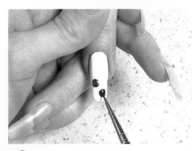

3 Dab a ball of glitter dust near the tip, and "twirl" it to form the first cherry. Wipe the brush clean. Make the second cherry.

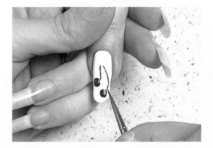

4 Mix and apply the green glitter dust, and drag it to form the stems.

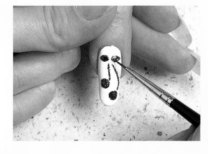

5 Mix and apply more green glitter dust. Tease the balls in to leaf-shapes. When dry, apply a coat of clear nail polish.

Bands of gold

1. Apply a base coat and two coats of nail polish. Allow to dry. Use a striping brush to paint three or four broad, diagonal, white lines across the nail.

2. Mix the gold glitter dust, and dab it at the junction of the white lines and drag it along the middle of the first line. Wipe the brush clean. Repeat to paint thin gold lines on the remaining white lines.

3. When dry, protect your nail art with a coat of clear nail polish.

You will need: base coat, black nail polish, white acrylic nail paint, striping brush, gold glitter dust, special mixer varnish, fine-tip glitter brush, and clear nail polish.

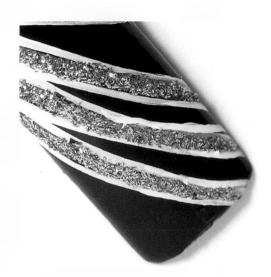

Rhinestone diamond

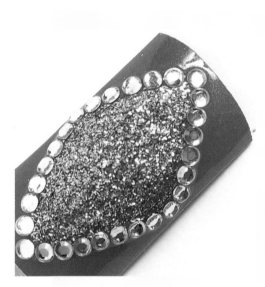

1. Apply a base coat and two coats of red nail polish, and allow to dry. Use a liner brush and gold acrylic nail paint to paint the diamond-shape.

2. Mix gold glitter dust and spread it to cover the diamond. It may take two or three applications. Allow to dry.

3. Apply clear nail varnish and use a dampened orangewood stick to position the rhinestones. Finish with clear nail varnish.

You will need: base coat, red nail polish, gold acrylic nail paint, liner brush, gold glitter dust, special mixer varnish, fine-tip glitter brush, rhinestones, orangewood stick, and clear nail polish.

Butterfly

1. Apply a base coat and two coats of base color nail polish, and allow to dry. Paint the butterfly using the art brush and black acrylic paint.

2. Use the method described in steps 2, 3, and 4 for "Stained glass" to mix and apply the glitter dust. Allow to dry.

3. Finish with two coats of clear nail varnish.

You will need: base coat; peach-colored nail polish; black acrylic nail paint; fine-tip art brush; gold, bronze (or orange), and silver glitter dust; special mixer varnish; fine-tip glitter brush; and clear nail polish.

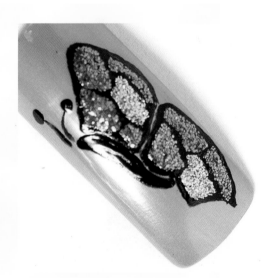

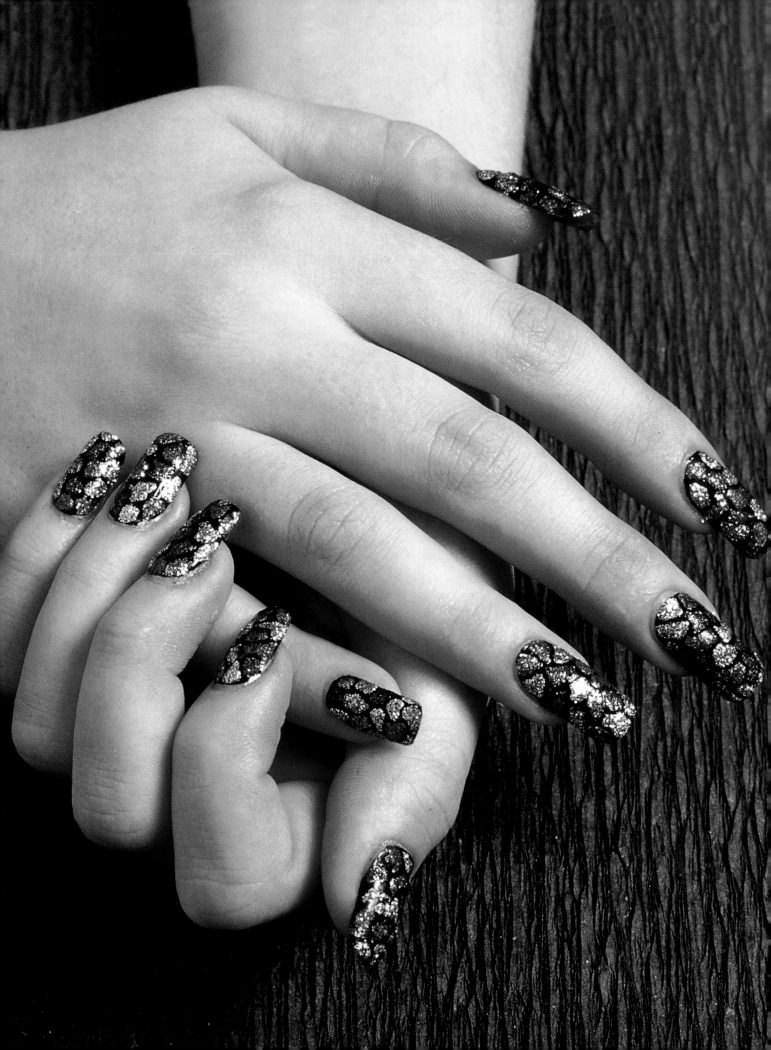

Embossed
Designs

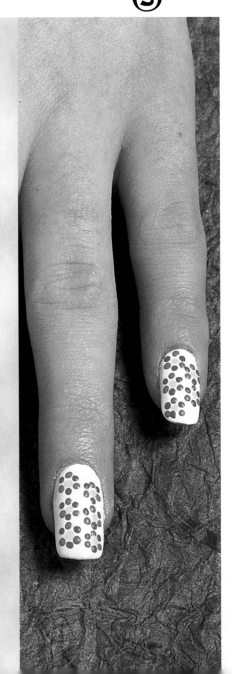

6

Embossed nail designs are created using a plastic, syringe-type tool filled with acrylic nail paint. When pressure is slowly applied to the plunger, the paint is forced out of the nozzle. To stop the flow of paint, release the pressure on the plunger. The technique is very similar to that used when decorating a cake. And like cake decoration, embossed designs are raised.

Two of the most comforting things about embossed nail art is that it requires no artistic flare –only three simple strokes are used–and success is assured. The three strokes used are: a dot, a line, and a "comma" shape. Combinations and simple variations on these three strokes, lets you paint everything from a swan to a spider web, a bow to a bouquet. Before you start nail painting, practise the basic strokes to get feel of the embossing tool and the flow of the paint.

The acrylic paint dries quite quickly, but you can speed up the process with warm air from a nail dryer or hair dryer. Acrylic paint does not dry to a glossy luster, so finish with a clear nail polish. To remove, use a conditioning nail polish remover.

Everything you need for embossed nail art is available in a kit. Kits usually contain a number of syringes, bottles of acrylic paint in various colors, a container, and a sponge. If you store your tools in the container, along with the damp sponge, the paint will remain moist and ready for use. Additional syringes and bottles of paint can be bought separately.

All-over design

This embossed design is perfect for novice nail artists as it uses only dots and "comma" strokes, and it can be simplified to suit your ability.

You will need:

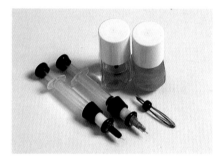

- base coat
- pink nail polish
- white and yellow paints
- embossing tools
- clear nail polish

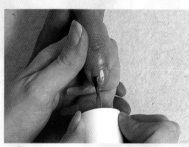

1 Apply a base coat and two coats of nail polish and allow to dry thoroughly.

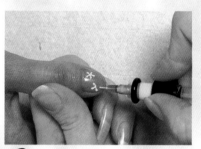

2 Use the yellow embossing tool to draw the flowers, using extended "commas". Paint incomplete "flowers" at the sides and tip.

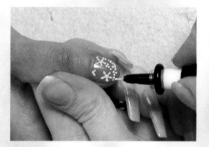

3 Add a shower of small dots with the white emboss tool. When the paint is dry, apply two coats of clear nail polish.

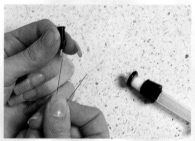

4 Should the nozzle of the embossing tool become blocked or the flow uneven, remove the nozzle and clean with a fine wire.

Be creative!

Nail art is a creative process—there are no hard and fast rules. The designs and colors suggested here are only a starting point. Designs can be simplified or made more complex, or elements from different designs merged to create something totally new. You may also want to personalize your nail art to incorporate your initials, or choose colors to match an outfit.

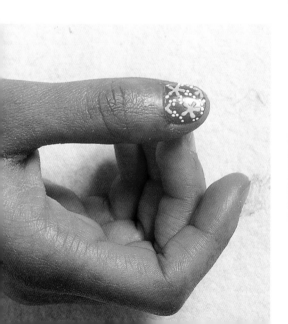

Swanning around

Though it may look complicated, this swan, gliding among reeds, is painted using "comma" shapes and a combination of curved and zigzag lines.

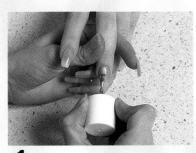

1 Apply a base coat and two coats of nail polish, and allow to dry thoroughly.

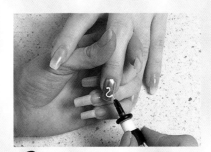

2 Use the white emboss tool to paint a "comma" for the swan's head. Continue the stroke, using a backward "S" for the neck and body.

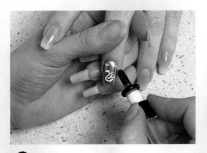

3 Stay with the white emboss tool and paint long "commas" for the wings, and "V" shapes for the birds.

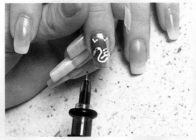

4 To make the beak, place the orange emboss tool close to the head and paint a "comma". Use black to form the eye.

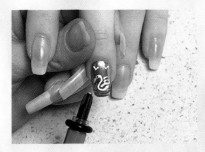

5 Paint lines across the nail, using the blue emboss tool, for the water. Add reeds with the green emboss tool. Finish with clear nail polish.

You will need:

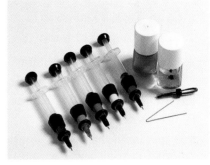

- base coat
- frosted, light blue nail polish
- white, orange, black, blue, and green paints
- embossing tools
- clear nail polish

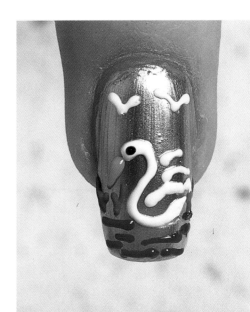

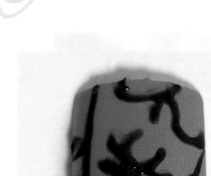

Spooky!

1. Apply a base coat and two coats of nail polish. Allow to dry.

2. Starting from a corner near the cuticle, use the black embossing tool to draw diagonal lines across the nail. Leave a space near the tip for the spider.

3. Link the diagonals with curved lines. The spider is based on "comma" shapes. When dry, apply two coats of clear nail polish.

You will need: base coat, pink nail polish, black paint, embossing tool, and clear nail polish.

Paws for thought

1. Apply a base coat and two coats of nail polish. Allow to dry.

2. Make the paw pads by drawing a circle with the black embossing tool, and then filling it in. Use dots for the claws.

3. When dry, "paws" for thought and don't forget to apply two coats of clear nail polish.

You will need: base coat, white nail polish, black paint, embossing tool, and clear nail polish.

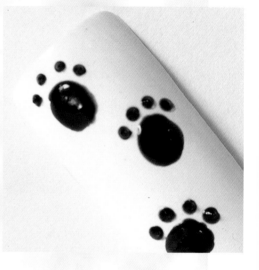

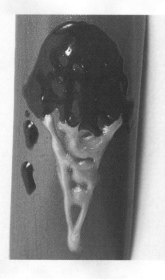

Strawberry sundae

1. Apply a base coat and two coats of nail polish. Allow to dry.

2. With the white embossing tool, draw the "V" of the cone. Use a wiggly line to lightly fill it in and give texture. Draw the outline of the dome-shaped, ice cream with the red embossing tool.

3. Fill in the outline and use "comma" shapes for the dripping ice cream. When dry, apply two coats of clear nail polish.

You will need: base coat, orange nail polish, white and red paints, embossing tools, and clear nail polish.

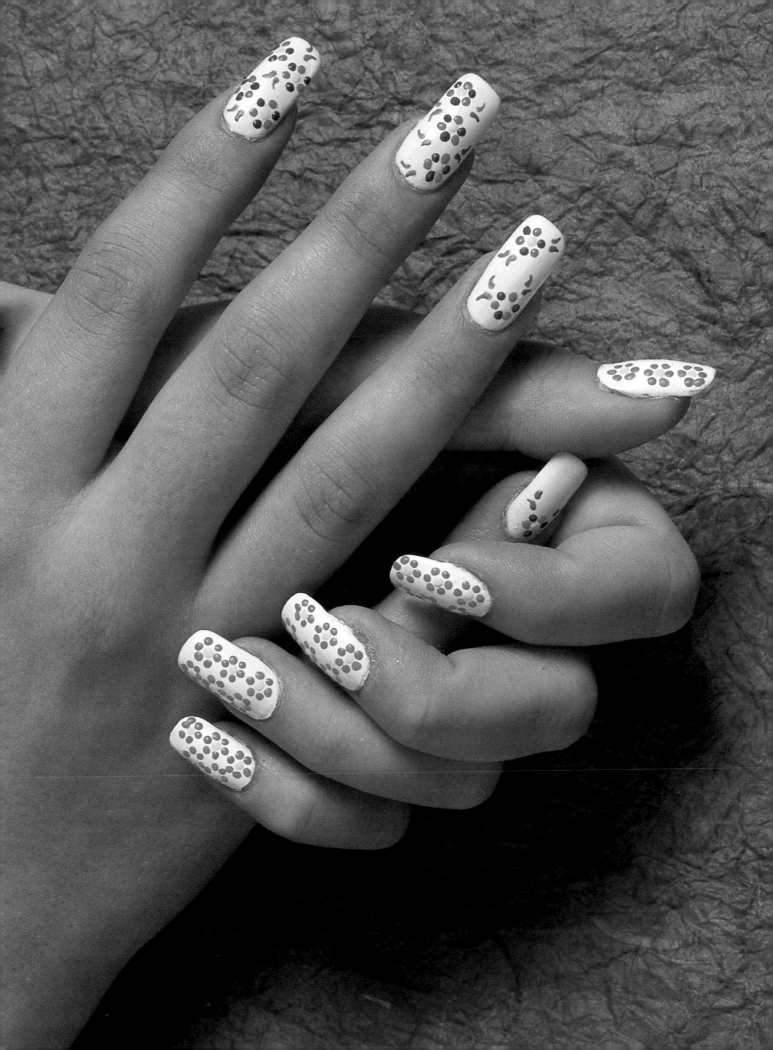

Party balloons

In this step-by-step, you will see how easy it is to give depth to a simple design using embossing tools. The white highlights make the balloons appear rounded.

You will need:

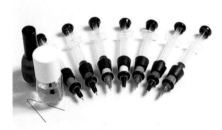

- base coat
- indigo nail polish
- pink, red, orange, yellow, blue, green, and white paints
- embossing tools
- clear nail polish

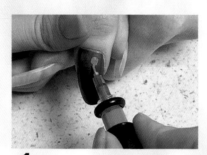

1 Apply a base coat and two coats of nail polish, and allow to dry thoroughly.

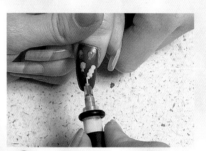

2 Draw the outlines of the pink, red, and orange balloons, then fill them in. Paint a small, triangle at the bottom of each balloon.

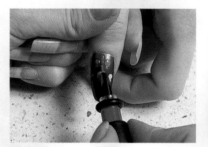

3 Form the long, yellow balloon with dots, and link them by using the nozzle like a "pen" to manipulate the acrylic paint.

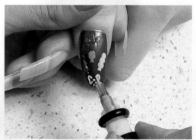

4 Fill spaces with blue and green balloons. Using the yellow embossing tool, draw fines lines to create the bow.

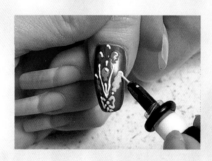

5 When the paint is dry, use the white embossing tool to draw strings from the balloons to the bow, and to paint highlights. Allow to dry, then apply two coats of clear nail polish.

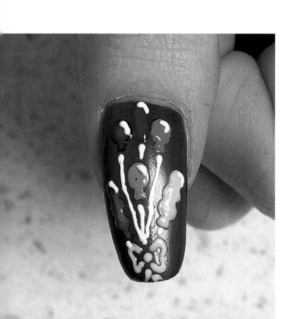

Racy stripes

1. Apply a base coat and two coats of nail polish. Allow to dry.

2. Use the embossing tool to draw three, very fine, broken lines diagonally across the nail. Keep them straight and parallel.

3. Fill each space with a dot (or a polish-secure rhinestone). When dry, apply clear nail polish.

You will need: base coat, blue nail polish, yellow paint, embossing tool, and clear nail polish.

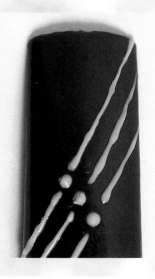

Snowdrop

1. Apply a base coat and two coats of nail polish. Allow to dry.

2. Using the green embossing tool, draw the stem finishing near the near the nail tip. Draw the outline and spines of the leaves.

3. Draw four "comma" shapes with the white embossing tool to create the dainty snowdrops. Allow to dry before applying two coats of clear nail polish.

You will need: base coat, red nail polish, green and white paints, embossing tools, and clear nail polish.

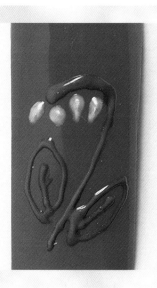

Sweetheart bow

1. Apply a base coat and two coats of nail polish. Allow to dry.

2. Draw a dot–almost in the center of the nail–then draw the outline shape of the bow. Add the dangling ribbons and detail inside the bow.

3. Draw a fine diagonal line either side of the bow. When dry, apply two coats of clear nail polish.

You will need: base coat, pink nail polish, yellow paint, embossing tool, and clear nail polish.

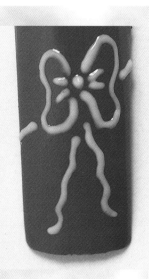

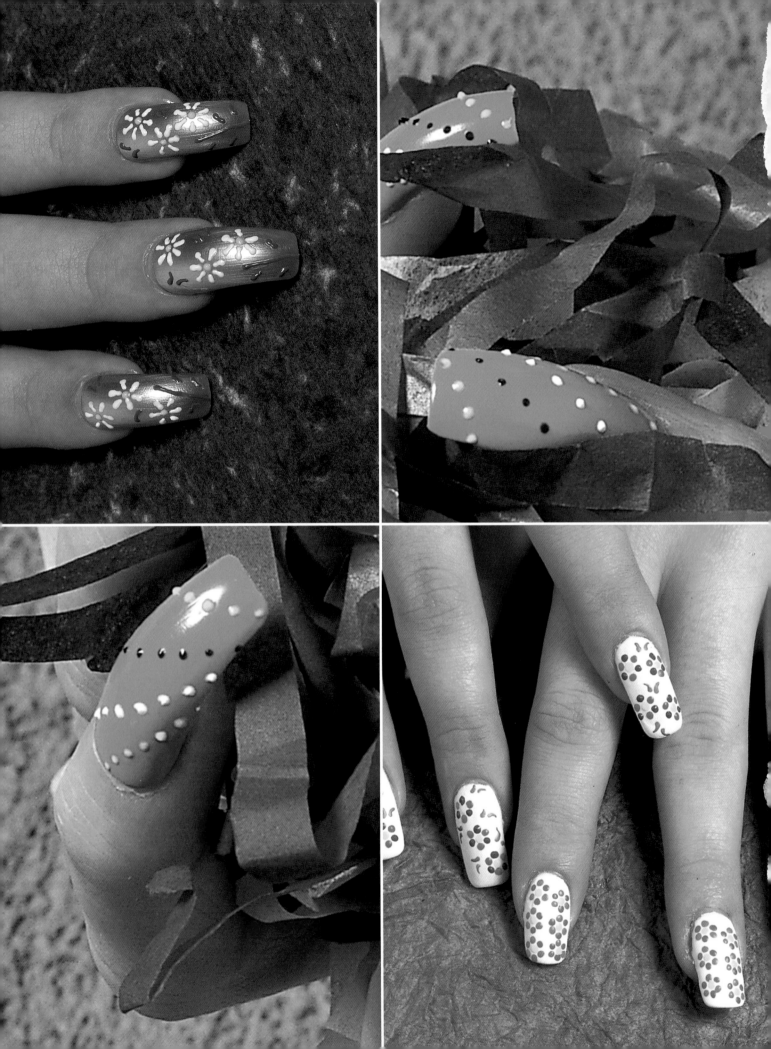

7
Paint
and Polish

Quick! Think of your favorite colors and then dream up some wacky patterns. Decorating your nails with paint and polish is that easy–and an original masterpiece is guaranteed every time.

There is only one limit to painting your nails in this way, and that's your imagination. So let yourself go. Over the next few pages we give you plenty of ideas, but really it is down to you what you do. The techniques used are the same and there are some crafty tools you can use to produce spectacular results.

Try to create color blends and contrasts that really work well together. Don't try to mix too many different colors together. You can use acrylic nail paint, opalescent paint, or nail polish. Opalescent paint is white, but when used sparingly over dark nail polish or acrylic paint it becomes iridescent.

An opalescent finish on black polish looks startling, while on purple, deep blue, or dark browns the result is stunning. On light colors, an opalescent top-coat gives an effect similar to mother of pearl–great for bridal designs. Practise with opalescent paint before using it. Paint it onto black

paper to see the effect it creates. If your masterpiece doesn't look right, don't despair–a clear top coat will bring the colors alive.

What tools to use? Brushes, obviously. You need a fine-tip art brush for detailed work, a fan brush for dragging designs, and a liner brush for thicker lines and for filling in larger areas with paint. There is also a striping brush, with long bristles, used for fine, long lines.

Other useful kit includes a marbling tool for dotting or swirling your paint or varnish. "Color Shaper" tools each have a differently shaped rubber end that achieve an endless assortment of patterns.

A neat trick is to use a stencil. Cut a tiny shape–a heart, stars, or moon–out of clear adhesive plastic and press it onto a pale-colored polished nail (but only when the polish is dry!). Then varnish over with your darker colors, and when dry remove the stencil with tweezers.

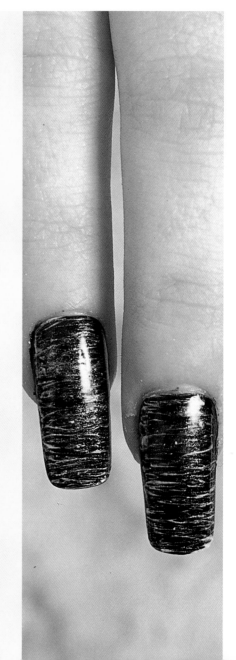

Marbling

Unless you are using a nail polish color that contrasts dramatically with the nail paint colors, the best marbling effect is achieved over a clear base coat. To prevent paint colors staining each other, apply tiny amounts each color onto a palette, and wipe the marbling tool clean when changing colors.

You will need:

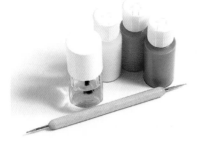

- clear base coat
- yellow, red, and neon blue acrylic nail paint
- paint palette or similar
- marbling tool
- paper towel
- clear nail polish

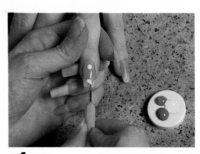

1 Apply a clear base coat. Use the larger round end of the marbling tool to drop blobs of yellow and red down the middle of the nail.

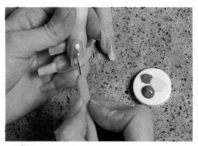

2 Wipe the marbling tool, then add blobs of neon blue to the nail. Don't worry if the colors start to blend on the nail.

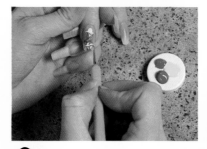

3 Wipe the marbling tool and use quick "comma" type stokes to swirl the colors together.

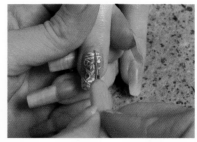

4 Continue marbling until the nail is covered. When dry apply two coats of clear nail polish.

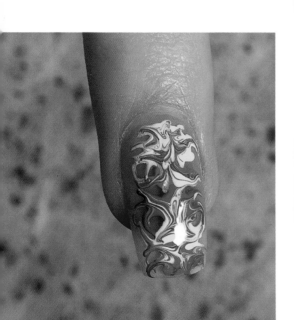

The light touch

Do not go overboard with the marbling tool and "swirl" the paints to a uniform muddy-brown color. The idea is to keep the colors distinct. Each time, before you let the marbling tool touch the paints, look critically at how the design is building up and how the colors are blending. The lightest and fastest of touches is all that is required to create the marbled look.

It's a gas!

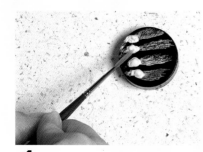

1 Even though opalescent paints appear white, their glorious colors become evident when they are applied in a thin film.

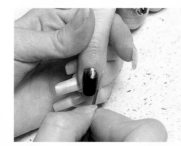

2 Apply a base coat and two coats of black nail polish. Allow to dry. Apply a thin film of gold opalescent paint near the cuticle using quick, diagonal strokes.

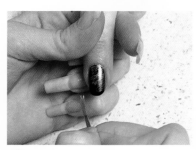

3 Apply green, blue, and violet in the same way, keeping the strokes diagonal and with bands of color building toward the nail tip.

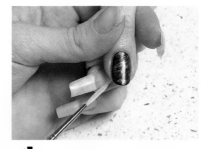

4 Merge the bands of colors by stroking the clean brush tip across the nail. When dry, apply two coats of clear nail polish.

If you've ever seen a pool of oil or gas and admired it's swirling patterns of colors, then you'll know the desired end-result of this paint and polish technique. This design is perfect for day- and evening-wear.

You will need:

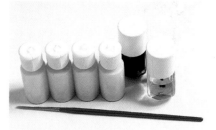

- base coat
- black nail polish
- blue, green, gold, and violet opalescent paints
- liner brush or fine-tip art brush
- paper towel
- clear nail varnish

Top tip

To achieve the iridescent effect, the opalescent paint must be applied in a very thin film. The best to way to guarantee this is to wipe all but the smallest amount of paint off the brush before you start your nail art. Remove excess paint by simply sweeping the brush back and forth on paper towel.

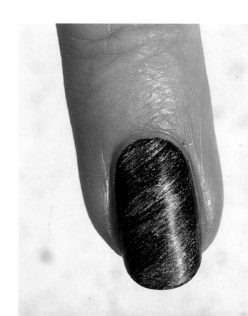

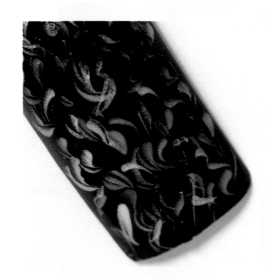

Confetti

1. Apply a base coat and two coats of nail polish. Allow to dry. Put small amounts of opalescent paints onto a palette.

2. Lightly dip the fine point of the "Taper-point tool" into gold opalescent paint. Wipe off any excess paint (see "Top tip", page 67).Using quick strokes to paint swirls all over the nail.

3. Repeat for the remaining colors, allowing the paint to dry between colors. Finish with two coats of clear nail polish.

You will need: base coat; black nail polish; gold, green, blue, and purple opalescent paints; "Taper-point tool"; palette; paper towel; and clear nail polish.

Shock waves

1. Apply a base coat and two coats of nail polish. Allow to dry. Put small amounts of opalescent paints onto a palette.

2. Lightly dip the "Angle chisel tool" into violet opalescent paint and drag the sharp edge of the tool across the nail. You need only the smallest amount of paint to create a stunning effect.

3. Allow the opalescent paint to dry before repeating with the remaining colors. Finish with a coat of clear nail polish.

You will need: base coat; purple nail polish; gold, green, blue, and violet opalescent paints; "Angle chisel tool"; palette; paper towel; and clear nail polish.

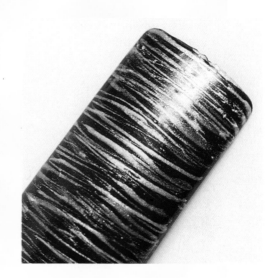

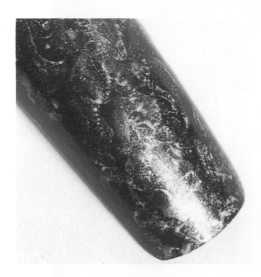

Dab-a-doo

1. Apply a base coat and two coats of nail polish. Allow to dry. Put small amounts of opalescent paints onto a palette.

2. Lightly dip the "Cup round tool" into violet opalescent paint, and dab the tool over the nail. Make sure the tool carries the barest amount of paint.

3. Allow to dry before repeating with the remaining color. Protect your nail art with a coat of clear nail polish.

You will need: base coat, red nail polish, violet and gold opalescent paints, "Cup round tool", palette, and clear nail polish.

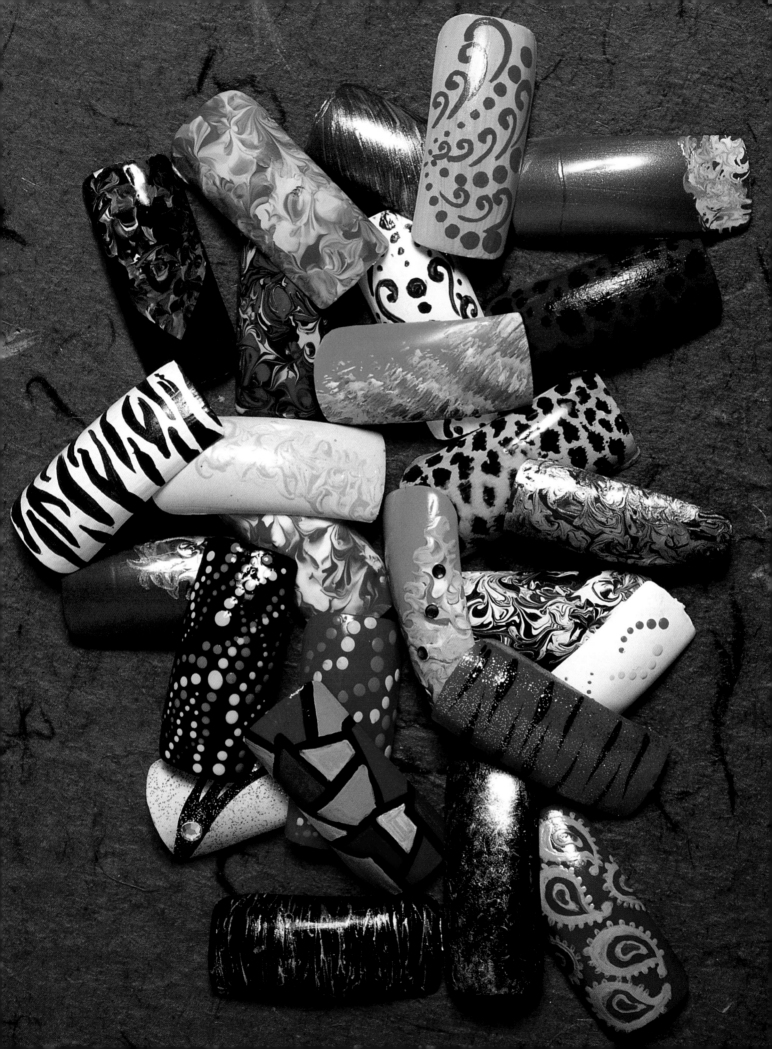

Fanfare

Ever so easy to do, but as in other paint and polish designs, less is often best. So that the wispy-effect is achieved, make sure the fan brush is not overloaded with paint. You can remove any excess by simply painting a few strokes onto paper towel.

You will need:

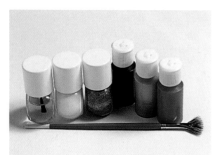

- base coat
- white nail polish
- red, black, and gold acrylic paints
- fan brush
- palette
- gold sparkle nail polish
- clear nail polish

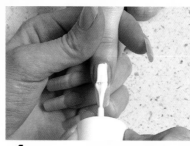

1 Apply a base coat and two coats of white nail polish, and allow to dry.

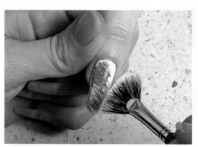

2 Put small amounts of each paint onto a palette. Dab the fan brush into the red nail paint. Wisp the brush lightly and diagonally across the nail.

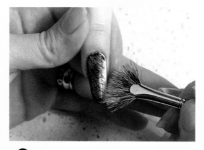

3 Repeat with the black nail paint, but make the diagonal sweep shorter so that a "fringe" of red is visible. When dry, apply the gold paint in the same way.

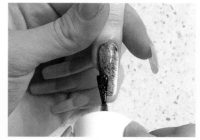

4 Add depth to the design with a coat of gold sparkle nail polish. When dry, protect your fanfare of nail art with one or two coats of clear nail polish.

Demure and dainty

A more subtle version of the dramatic "Fanfare" can be created by painting shades of cream, pink and peach over the white base color. Use the same technique, keeping the strokes diagonal and light. Finish with clear nail polish suspended with dots or strands of silver glitter.

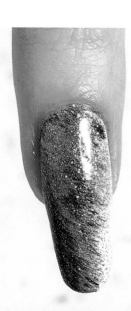

Going dotty

1. Apply a base coat and two coats of nail polish, and allow to dry.

2. Dip the tool into red nail paint. Dab it on the nail to make the dots. As the paint runs out, the dots will decrease in size. Repeat for the remaining colors to create a random pattern.

3. Allow to dry before applying two coats of clear nail polish.

You will need: base coat; white nail polish; yellow, orange, pink, red, green, and blue neon nail paint; "Taper-point tool" or marble tool; palette; paper towel; and clear nail polish.

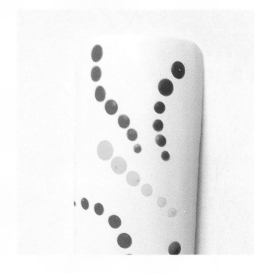

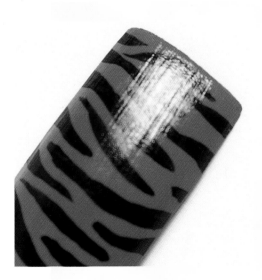

Tiger, tiger

1. Apply a base coat and two coats of nail polish. Allow to dry.

2. Using the brush and black nail paint, paint a short wavy line halfway across the nail near the nail tip. Apply further strokes, vary the line's thickness and shape from outside edge to middle.

3. Using the same technique, create a tiger pattern over the nail. Allow to dry, then finish with two coats of clear nail polish.

You will need: base coat, orange nail polish, black nail paint, fine-tip art brush, and clear nail polish.

Leopard spots

1. Apply a base coat and two coats of nail polish, and allow to dry.

2. Use the brush and light brown paint to draw eight to ten circles on the nail. Dab the brush to blur the edges of the circles.

3. Cover the nail and fill the circles with tiny "smudges" of light brown paint. When dry, apply two coats of clear nail polish.

You will need: base coat, cream nail polish, light brown nail paint, fine-tip art brush, and clear nail polish.

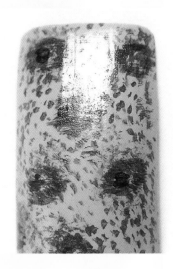

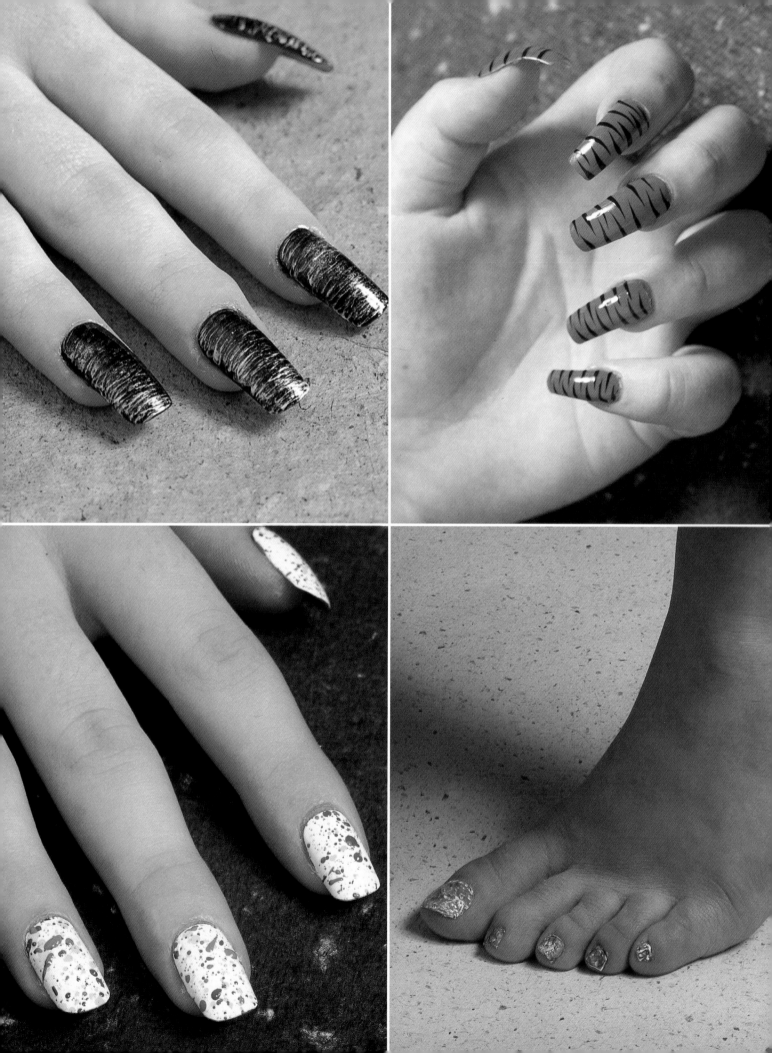

8

Hands-on
Nail Art

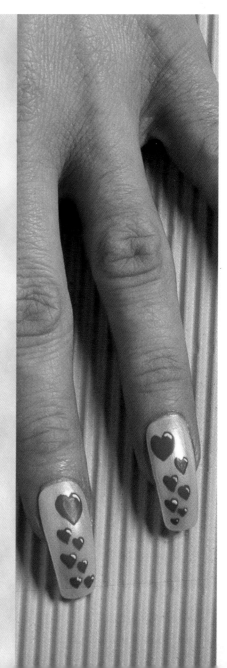

Hand-drawing your own pictures on your nails is difficult, right? It can be, but it doesn't have to be. So keep reading!

Many of the designs we show you here were drawn by professional nail artists, but some of the simpler designs were painted by nail art fans on their first attempts. Nail pictures don't have to be complex, and very often the simplest are the most effective. This is also a good nail art technique to master because a hand-drawn picture can be made to suit–even flatter–any nail shape or length.

There are many brands of acrylic paint available and most will be suitable for painting nails. If in doubt, ask your nail product retailer. The brushes are cleaned by simply washing in warm, soapy water, rinsing, and then drying with paper towel.

One thing for sure about hand-drawing your own designs–if you keep them simple and the colors bold, you are sure to surprise yourself at how professional the finished picture looks. You never know, you may discover a hidden talent and a whole new career as a professional nail artist may open up! If you are that good and want to take it further, nail product retailers and some colleges hold training courses in exactly this field.

Parrot fashion

This crazy parrot could be your first nail art creation. There's no harm in practising painting the shapes on paper first to refine your skill and perfect the lines. But don't be tempted to draw it larger, nail art requires the skill of a miniaturist.

You will need:

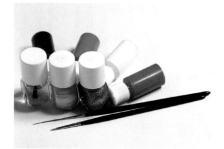

- base coat
- silver nail polish
- red, white, green, and black acrylic paints
- fine-tip and liner brushes
- palette
- sparkle nail polish
- clear nail polish

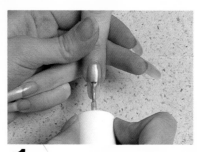

1 Apply a base coat and two coats of silver nail polish. Allow to dry. Put small amounts of the acrylic paints onto a palette.

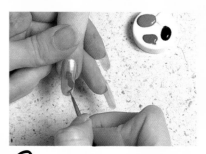

2 Use the fine-tip brush and red paint to paint the parrot–its head is in the center of the nail. Paint fine lines for the head feathers.

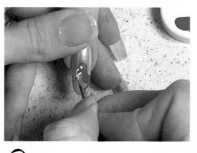

3 Allow to dry before painting the beak, wing, and eye with white paint.

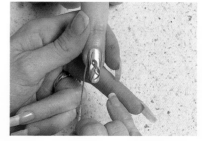

4 Paint, using the liner brush, fine green lines to create the branches of the tree.

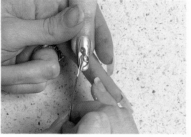

5 Paint white highlights to one side of the branches and define the wing. Apply sparkle polish to the wing. Paint a black dot in the center of the eye. Finish with two coats of clear nail polish.

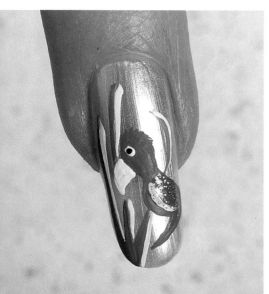

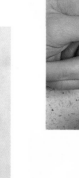

Palm tree

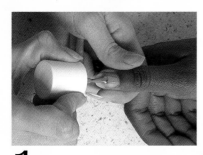

1 Apply a base coat and two coats of orange nail polish. Allow to dry. Put small amounts of the acrylic paints onto a palette.

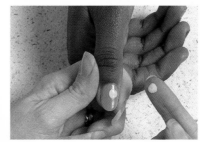

2 Dip a fingertip in the yellow paint, then press it lightly onto the nail for the moon. Allow to dry.

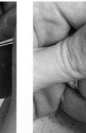

3 Paint, using the side of a striping brush, fine black lines halfway across the nail near the tip for the sea. Let the last line sweep upward.

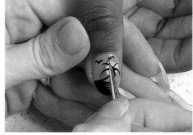

4 Continue with the black to paint the branches on the palm tree and seagulls. Do this with the fine-tip brush.

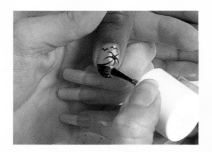

5 When the paint is dry, apply silver sparkle nail polish over the nail tip. Finish with one or two coats of clear nail polish

What a way to remember to wonderful tropical holiday or, better still, to drop a subtle hint for a holiday destination. When you become more confident with your painting skills, add another palm tree, but make it smaller so that it appears further away.

You will need:

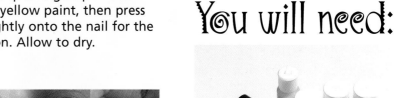

- base coat
- orange nail polish
- yellow and black acrylic paints
- fine-tip and striping brush
- palette
- silver sparkle nail polish
- clear nail polish

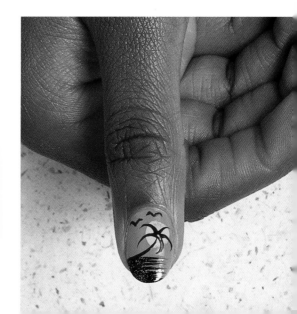

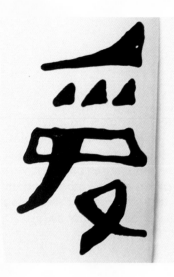

Chinese character

1. Apply a base coat and two coats of white nail polish. Allow to dry. The character you are going to write means "love".

2. Using the brush and black paint, copy the shapes in the picture. Where necessary, draw an outline of the shape and then fill it in.

3. When the paint is dry, apply two coats of clear nail polish.

You will need: base coat, white nail polish, black acrylic paint, fine-tip art brush, and clear nail polish.

Indian aum

1. Apply a base coat and two coats of pale blue nail polish. Allow to dry. The word aum means "sounds of the Earth".

2. Using the brush and purple paint, first paint the figure resembling a "3", then add the final two strokes and a dot.

3. When the paint is dry apply two coats of clear nail polish.

You will need: base coat, pale blue nail polish, purple acrylic paint, fine-tip art brush, and clear nail polish.

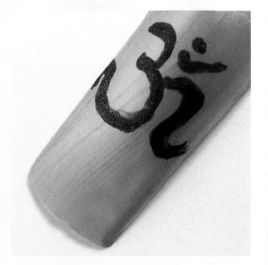

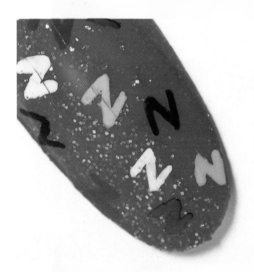

From A to Z

1. Apply a base coat and two coats of nail polish. Allow to dry. You can decorate your nail with any combination of letters you like.

2. Paint capital letters all over the nail in a random pattern using the five paints and brush. When dry, apply sparkle nail polish.

3. Finish with one coat of protective clear nail polish.

You will need: base coat; pink nail polish; green, red, white, blue, and yellow acrylic paints; gold sparkle nail polish; fine-tip art brush; and clear nail polish.

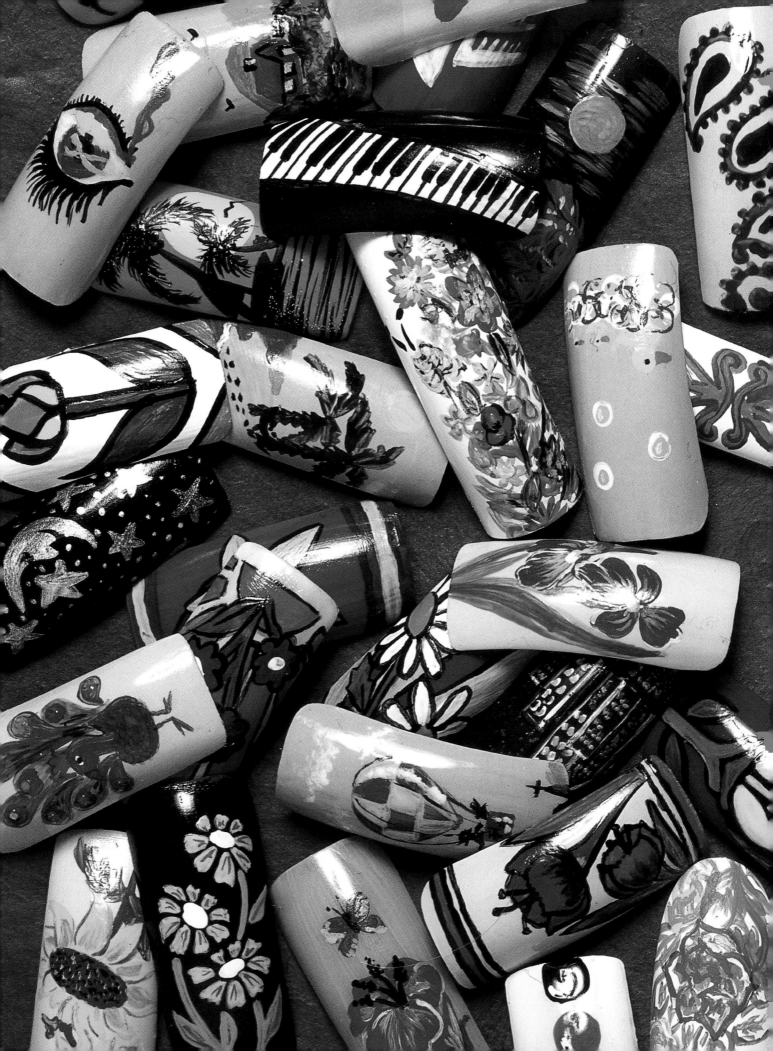

Flower power

This is a great favorite with young children and teenagers. You can paint the petals to match their outfit and give each flower a different expression.

You will need:

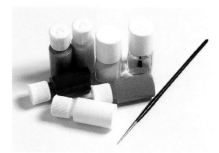

- base coat
- yellow, orange, green, white, and black acrylic paints
- fine-tip art brush
- palette
- clear nail polish

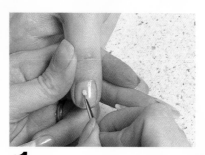

1 Apply two layers of base coat, and allow to dry. Put small amounts of the paints onto a palette. Paint a yellow circle in the center of the nail.

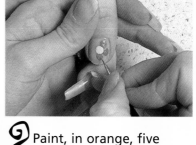

2 Paint, in orange, five petals around the center.

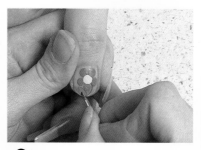

3 Paint a stem running to the nail tip and two leaves in green paint.

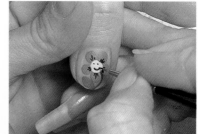

4 Use white paint to create eyes, then add details in black paint. When dry, apply two coats of clear nail polish.

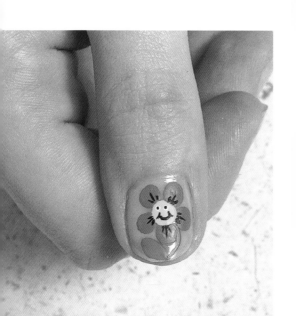

Eye for detail

Even though these hand-painted artworks are in miniature, they do benefit from the inclusion of some detail. To include every nuance would be impossible, so be selective. For such detailed work, a quality fine-tip art brush is a big advantage. Care for the brush by washing and rinsing it after use, and drying the bristles gently to a fine point. Stand the brush, bristles-up, in a container ready for use.

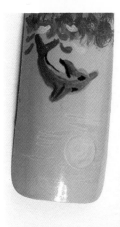
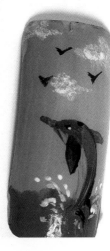

Dolphin watch

1. Apply a base coat and two coats of blue nail polish. Allow to dry. Use the brush and blue paint to paint waves at the nail tip. Allow each color to dry before applying the next.

2. Paint the dolphin using shades of gray paint, then add black shading and a white dot for the eye. Continue with the white paint to create clouds and water splash.

3. Fill the sky with birds or a golden sun. When dry, apply two coats of clear nail polish.

You will need: base coat; sky-blue nail polish; gray, black, white, dark blue, and yellow acrylic paints; fine-tip art brush; and clear nail polish.

New York, New York

1. Apply a base coat and two coats of blue nail polish. Allow to dry. Paint the moon and the birds, white.

2. Paint part of the nail tip black, as shown. Still using black paint, draw vertical lines for the buildings. Outline the buildings in white and draw the horizon. Use quick strokes of white paint to add texture to the water

3. Paint glitter polish onto the buildings, and apply silver sparkle polish to the nail tip. When dry, finish with clear nail polish.

You will need: base coat, silvery-blue nail polish, white and black acrylic paints, fine-tip art brush, glitter nail polish, silver sparkle nail polish and clear nail polish.

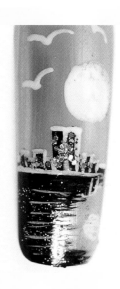

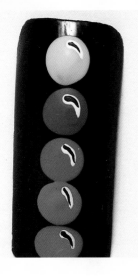

Stop 'n' go

1. Apply a base coat and two coats of nail polish. Allow to dry.

2. Use the brush to dab a small blob of yellow near the tip. Press lightly with the tip of a finger to form a circle. Repeat the technique with the remaining colors, allowing the paint to dry before starting on the next color.

3. Highlight each circle with black over white paint. When dry, apply two coats of clear nail polish.

You will need: base coat; black nail polish; yellow, blue, pink, green, and orange neon acrylic paints; fine-tip art brush; white and black paints, and clear nail polish.

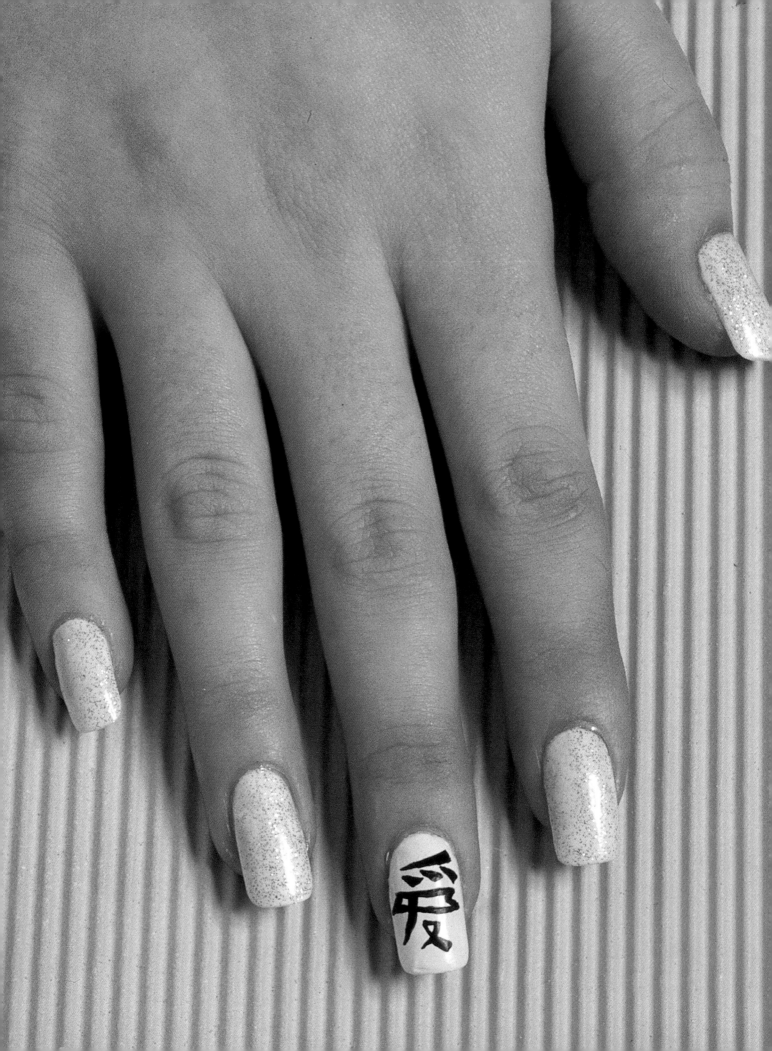

Foil Designs

The effect achieved with foil cannot be replicated by any other type of polish or paint, stick-on or stencil. There's something specially startling about the way the multi-colored or patterned, wafer-thin foil catches the light as your hands move. The cracked, almost antique-effect, that can be created with unadorned gold and silver foil is one to behold.

You can buy foil on a roll or in sheets, and it consists of a colored metallic foil bonded to a clear backing. When the foil–silver-side down–comes in contact with a special cold-release adhesive painted onto the nail, the foil sticks to the nail while the backing peels off. The foil backing can be peeled off the nail almost immediately after you've completed rubbing the foil with a cotton bud.

As the foil will only stick to the adhesive, it is important you apply the glue exactly where you want it. After using the glue brush or an art brush to paint on the adhesive, wash it in soapy water. On application, cold-release adhesive is opaque. When it becomes clear, it is time to position the foil on the nail and rub to assure contact.

Never apply the cold-release adhesive to a bare nail. The oils in natural nails will reduce the bonding between the foil and the adhesive. Protect natural nails and improve the finish of foil nail art by using a quality base coat under a nail polish color similar to the foil. The nail polish color will then conceal any tears or gaps in the foil.

Foil is extremely thin, so protect it with clear nail polish, and routinely apply further top coats every other day.

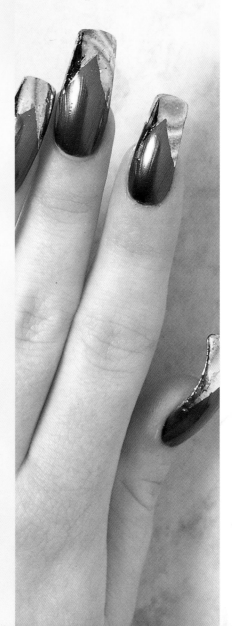

Polka dots

Starting with this dotty design, gives you the opportunity to become familiar with working with foil and the adhesive, yet at the same time create a delightful piece of nail art. When you feel more confident, go onto covering an entire nail, as shown on the next page.

You will need:

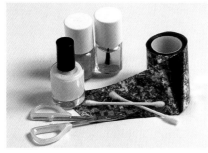

- base coat
- pink nail polish
- roll of multi-colored foil
- scissors
- cold-release adhesive
- cotton buds
- clear nail polish

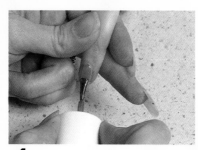

1 Apply a base coat and two coats of pink nail polish, and allow to dry.

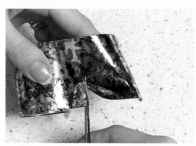

2 Cut a rectangle of foil large enough to cover the nail and easy to handle.

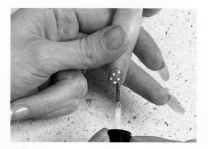

3 Apply dots of adhesive all over the nail using the brush. When first applied, the adhesive will be white.

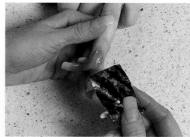

4 When the adhesive becomes clear, lay the foil –silver-side down, colored surface face up–onto the nail.

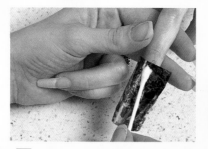

5 Rub a cotton bud gently over the foil to make sure that it has made contact with the adhesive.

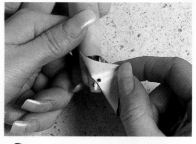

6 Lift the foil by the edge and peel it off to leave a thin coating of foil on the glue-covered areas. Apply two coats of clear nail varnish.

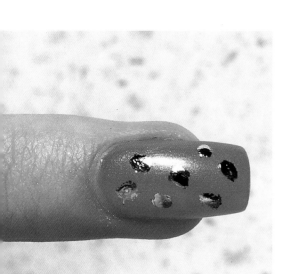

Mirage

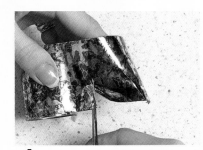

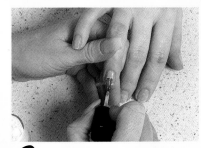

A spectacular nail art effect, but getting complete coverage requires a little practice. The wonderful thing about nail art, though, is that there is never a problem getting hold of volunteers happy to have their nails decorated!

1 Apply a base coat and two coats of nail polish, and allow to dry. Cut a rectangle of foil larger than the nail.

2 Apply adhesive to the whole nail, paying special attention to the edges. The adhesive will be white.

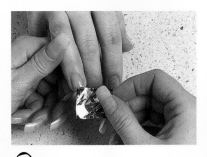

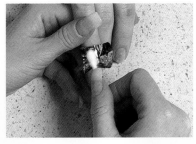

You will need:

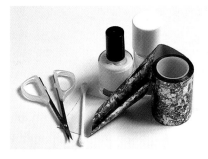

3 When the adhesive becomes clear, lay the foil –silver-side down, colored surface face up–onto the nail.

4 Rub a cotton bud over the foil, gently pressing it into the sides and over the free edge.

- base coat
- clear or colored nail polish
- clear nail polish
- roll of multi-colored foil
- scissors
- cold-release adhesive
- cotton bud

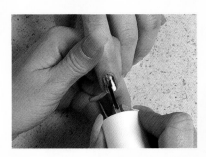

5 Lift the foil by the edge and peel away to leave the foil design. Protect with two coats of clear nail polish.

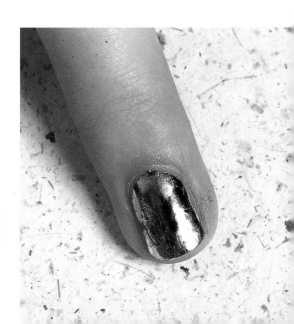

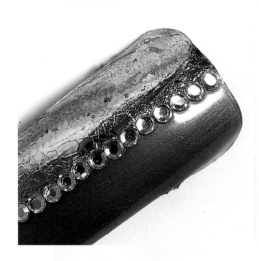

Split image

1. Apply a base coat and two coats of blue nail polish, and allow to dry. Apply adhesive to the right-hand side of the nail only.

2. When the adhesive becomes clear, lay a piece of foil–silver-side down–over the adhesive. Rub a cotton bud gently over the foil, then peel up the foil.

3. Apply a coat of clear nail polish over the whole nail. While wet, position rhinestones to conceal any flaws along the foil edge. Finish with another coat of clear nail polish.

You will need: base coat, electric blue nail polish, multi-colored foil, scissors, cold-release adhesive, cotton bud, clear nail polish, rhinestones, and an orangewood stick.

Carnival

1. Apply a base coat and two coats of yellow nail polish, and allow to dry. Paint a wiggly line and dot using the brush and adhesive.

2. When the adhesive becomes clear, lay the foil–silver-side down–over the whole nail. Rub a cotton bud gently over the foil.

3. Peel off the foil. Apply two coats of clear nail polish to finish.

You will need: base coat, yellow nail polish, multi-colored foil, scissors, cold-release adhesive, fine-tip art brush, cotton bud, and clear nail polish.

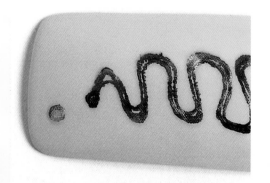

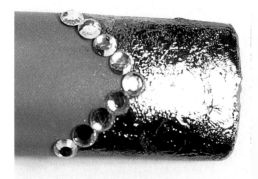

Chevron foil

1. Apply a base coat and two coats of lilac nail polish, and allow to dry. Apply adhesive sparingly to the nail tip in a chevron design.

2. When the adhesive becomes clear, lay the foil–silver-side down–over the whole nail. Rub a cotton bud gently over the foil. Peel off the foil backing.

3. Apply a coat of clear nail polish, and while wet, position rhinestones along "V" edge of the foil. Finish with another coat of clear nail polish.

You will need: base coat, lilac nail polish, multi-colored foil, scissors, cold-release adhesive, cotton bud, clear nail polish, rhinestones, and an orangewood stick.

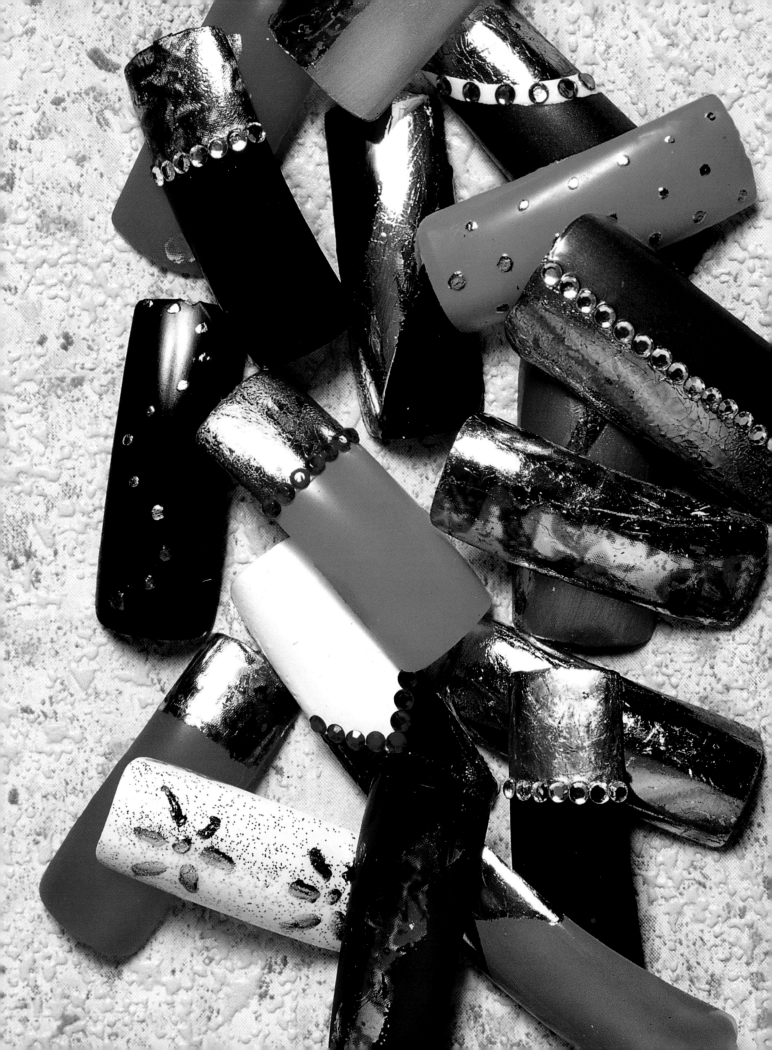

Foil flower

When applying the cold-release adhesive, use only the barest amount. If the adhesive is too thick, it will spread when the foil is rubbed onto the nail and any detail in your design will be lost.

You will need:

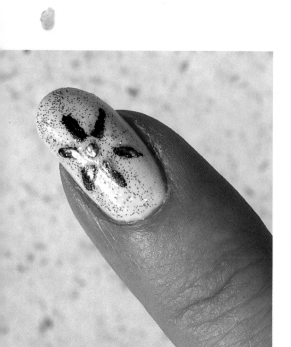

- base coat
- white nail polish
- multi-colored foil
- scissors
- fine-tip art brush
- cold-release adhesive
- cotton bud
- silver glitter nail polish
- clear nail polish

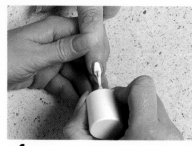

1 Apply a base coat and two coats of nail polish, and allow to dry. Cut a piece of foil larger than the nail.

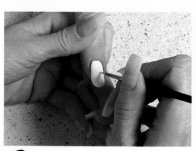

2 Use the tip of the brush to paint a dot and six radiating lines of adhesive.

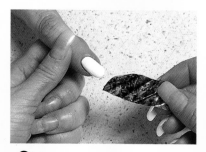

3 When the adhesive becomes clear, lay the foil –silver-side down–onto the nail.

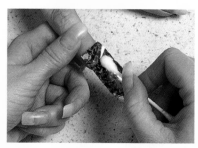

4 Rub a cotton wool bud gently over the foil to make sure that it has made contact with the adhesive.

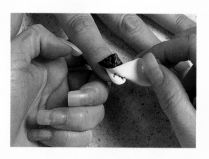

5 Lift off the foil by the edge and peel it away to leave a thin coating of foil on the glue-covered areas. Apply a coat of silver glitter nail polish. When dry follow with a coat of clear nail varnish.

Brushstrokes

1. Apply a base coat and two coats of red nail polish, and allow to dry. Cut a rectangle of foil, then paint three sweeping lines diagonally across the nail, as shown, using the brush and adhesive.

2. When the adhesive becomes clear, lay the foil–silver-side down–onto the nail. Rub a cotton wool bud gently over the foil.

3. Peel off the foil. Apply two coats of clear nail polish to finish.

You will need: base coat, red nail polish, gold foil, scissors, cold-release adhesive, art brush, cotton bud, and clear nail polish.

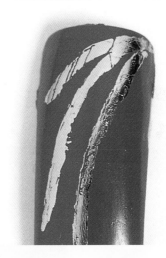

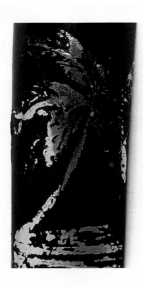

Palm d'Or

1. Apply a base coat and two coats of black nail polish, and allow to dry. Cut a rectangle of foil. Using the art brush and adhesive, paint horizontal lines across the nail tip for the water. Then go on to paint the tree and birds. Use the barest amount of adhesive.

2. When the adhesive becomes clear, lay the foil–matt silver-side down–onto the nail. Rub a cotton wool bud gently over the foil.

3. Peel off the foil. Apply two coats of clear nail polish to finish.

You will need: base coat, black nail polish, gold foil, scissors, cold-release adhesive, art brush, cotton bud, and clear nail polish.

Silver shield

1. Apply a base coat and two coats of black nail polish, and allow to dry. Cut a rectangle of foil. Paint a broad diagonal line of adhesive across the nail.

2. When the adhesive becomes clear, lay the foil–matt silver-side down–onto the nail. Rub a cotton wool bud gently over the foil. Peel off the foil.

3. Cut two lengths of striping tape, each slightly longer the nail. Position one along either edge of the foil. Smooth and trim. Protect your nail art with two coats of clear nail polish.

You will need: base coat, black nail polish, silver foil, scissors, cold-release adhesive, cotton bud, silver striping tape, and clear nail polish.

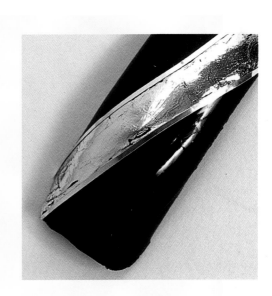

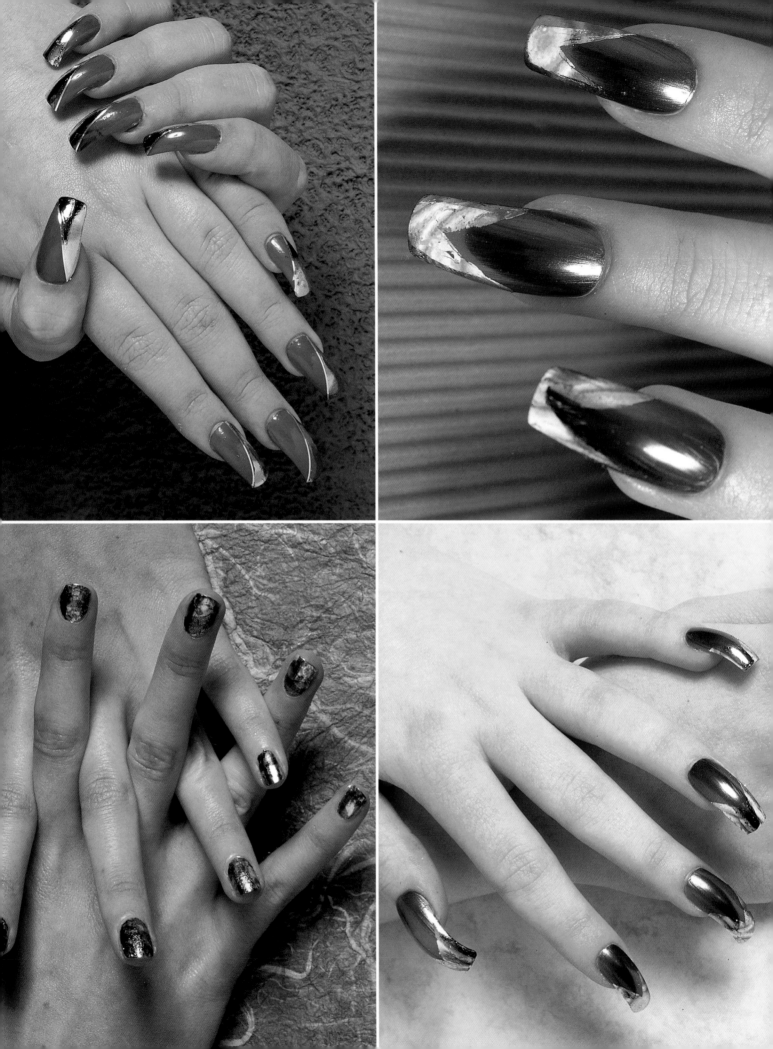

10

Airbrush
Nail Art

You can achieve subtle shades, blends of colors, and intricate designs with an airbrush that simply aren't possible with a normal brush.

What is an airbrush? It's a device that applies a water-based paint by blowing it onto the nail surface in a superfine spray. A dual-action airbrush allows you to control both color and air with one finger, and this is the type to go for. The air and paint are mixed together inside the airbrush to produce the fine spray–it uses only a few drops of paint and it dries in seconds.

The bad news is that an airbrush with its vital compressor isn't cheap, but there are lots of different types at different prices so they are worth checking out at your local nail art retailer–perhaps a group of friends could buy one together to share.

Apart from professional results, an airbrush also means you need never buy a bottle of colored nail polish again, since you can mix your own paint colors.

With masking film (called "Frisket" film) or stencils you can airbrush amazing geometric patterns. A stencil and airbrush are the easiest way to achieve the popular French nail designs and to create a detailed picture that is built up in sections. Your nails will look a million dollars, but don't try an airbrush design five minutes before a party! It takes time, practice, and patience.

When airbrushing, always use a quality clear base coat and finish with clear polish or nail art sealer. It's also important to understand how colors blend best. A good tip is to always spray white paint onto the base coat. This will give depth to colors and a smooth surface. Remember, yellow paint sprayed onto blue may give you green, so spray the yellow first, then the blue. It is inevitable that paint will spray onto the skin around the nail and onto the work surface. Don't worry, the water-based paint washes off easily.

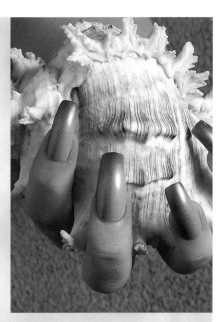

Airbrush care

To clean the airbrush between colors, place a few drops of airbrush cleaner into the cavity and spray excess paint through onto sheets of paper towel.

It is a good practice to leave a few drops of cleaner in the cavity when the airbrush is not in use. This will prevent any build-up, prior to a thorough and detailed clean following the manufacturer's instructions.

Tri-tone

This is the most subtle of airbrush designs where shades of color seamlessly change from dark to light. Move the airbrush swiftly back and forth over the nail to build up fine layers of paint. Moving the airbrush too slowly will create pools of uneven paint, which lack the distinctive texture of airbrush work.

You will need:

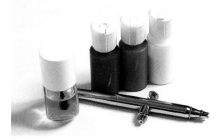

- base coat
- airbrush equipment and cleaner
- white, light blue, and dark blue paint
- clear nail polish
- cotton buds

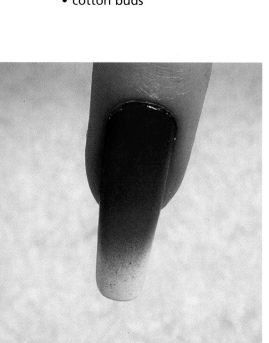

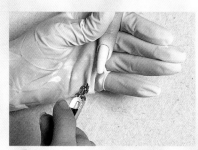

1 Apply a clear base coat and allow to dry. Airbrush the nail, white. Spray away excess color with cleaner (see page 89).

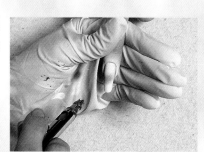

2 Spray a light blue diagonal band across the nail. Between every color-change, spray away excess paint with cleaner.

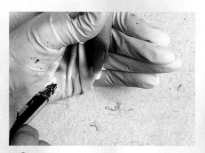

3 Spray the area between the light blue band and the cuticle, dark blue. Move the airbrush diagonally, not straight across the nail.

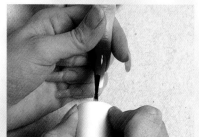

4 When dry, apply two coats of clear polish all over the nail.

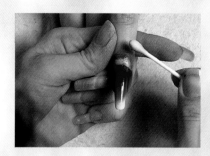

5 Remove overspray with warm, soapy water and a cotton bud. Clean the airbrush following the manufacturer's instructions.

Eye of the tiger

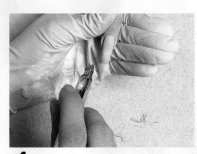

1 Apply a clear base coat. Airbrush the nail, white. Spray away excess paint with cleaner (see page 89), then spray the nail, fawn.

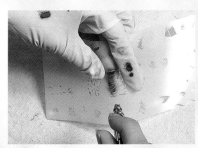

2 Before each color change, spray through with cleaner. Hold the tiger skin stencil firmly on the nail. Spray with black paint.

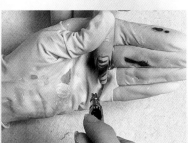
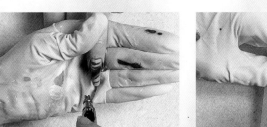

3 Remove the stencil carefully, and spray a diagonal black band across the middle of the nail.

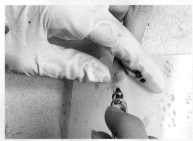

4 Firmly hold the almond-shaped stencil (the eye) in the middle of the black band, and spray with fawn paint. Remove the stencil.

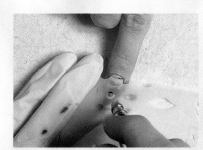

5 Place the small circular stencil (the pupil) at the top of the almond-shape and in the middle. Spray this stencil, black.

6 Place the crescent stencil over the iris, and spray it white. Remove and apply coats of clear nail polish. Use soapy water and cotton buds to remove overspray.

Airbrushing and stencils are natural partners. The fine spray of paint generated by the airbrush means that even tiny stencils are reproduced perfectly. This design is called a "build up" stencil design. It is a simple way of creating quite complicated scenes, images and characters. The final step is to clean your equipment thoroughly.

You will need:

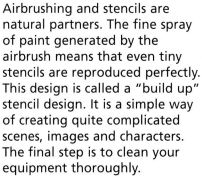

- clear base coat
- airbrush equipment and cleaner
- white, fawn, and black paint
- tiger skin stencil, and an "eye" stencil with almond (eye) and crescent (highlight) shapes, and a small circle (pupil)
- clear nail polish
- cotton buds

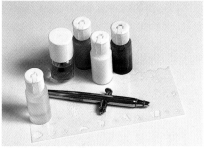
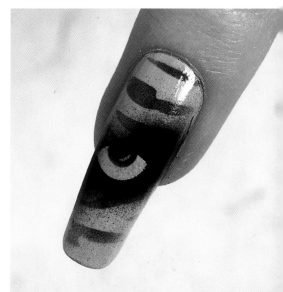

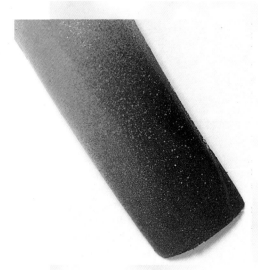

Duo-tone

1. Apply a clear base coat, and allow to dry. Airbrush the nail white. Spray away excess paint (see page 89) with cleaner before each color change.

2. Spray the nail lilac. Fill the airbrush with purple paint and, starting near the tip, spray two-thirds of the nail purple. Move the airbrush quickly and diagonally across the nail.

3. Apply two coats of clear nail polish and allow to dry. Remove the overspray with soapy water and cotton buds. Clean the airbrush following the manufacturer's instructions.

You will need: clear base coat; airbrush equipment and cleaner; white, lilac, and metallic purple paint; clear nail polish; and cotton buds.

Totally abstract

1. Apply a clear base coat, and allow to dry. Spray the nail white. Spray away excess paint (see page 89) with cleaner before every color change. Spray the nail with yellow, orange, and red paint following the instructions for "Tri-tone" on page 90.

2. Use the knife to cut triangles–without cutting the backing paper–from "Frisket" film. Peel off the shapes and press them onto the nail.

3. Spray the nail, black. When dry, carefully remove the triangles with tweezers. Apply coats of clear polish. Remove overspray with soapy water and cotton buds. Clean the airbrush thoroughly.

You will need: clear base coat; airbrush equipment and cleaner; white, yellow, orange, red, and black paint; "Frisket" film; craft knife; clear nail polish; and cotton buds.

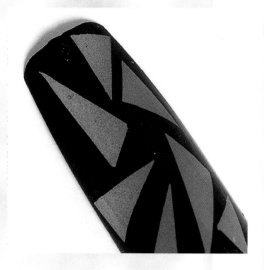

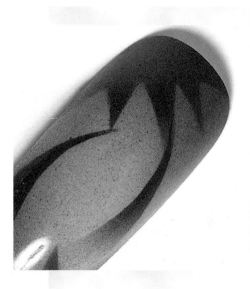

Jungle beat

1. Apply a clear base coat, and allow to dry. Spray the nail white. Spray away excess paint (see page 89) with cleaner before each color change. Spray diagonally opposite corners of the nail, light brown.

2. Spray a diagonal band across the center of the nail, light peach. Use the spike stencil and dark brown paint to decorate the light brown corners.

3. Stencil two large, single spikes in the middle of the nail using gray paint. Apply coats of clear. Remove overspray with soapy water and cotton buds. Clean the airbrush thoroughly.

You will need: clear base coat; airbrush equipment and cleaner; white, light brown, pale peach, dark brown, and gray paint; stencil; clear nail polish; and cotton buds.

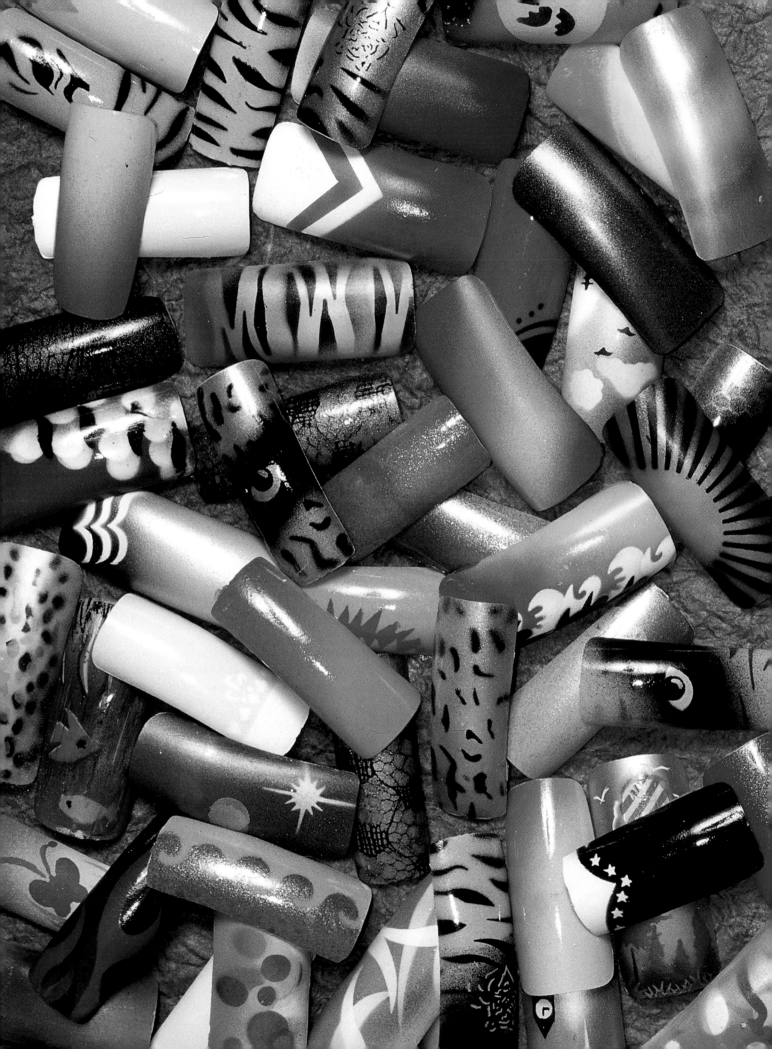

Frisket butterfly

"Frisket" film consists of a layer of clear adhesive plastic on a peel-off backing sheet. It can be used to create your own stencils using a cutter punch or a craft knife. The butterfly cutter punch is a very popular motif, and if you have long nails you may like to stencil it two or more times on each nail.

You will need:

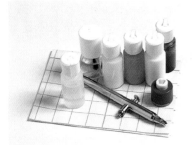

- clear base coat
- airbrush equipment and cleaner
- white, neon pink, neon yellow, and black paint
- butterfly cutter punch
- "Frisket" film
- clear nail polish
- cotton buds

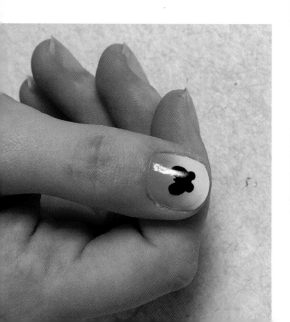

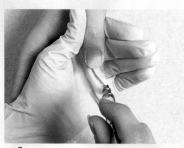

1 Apply a clear base coat and, when dry, spray the nail white. Spray away excess paint (see page 89) with cleaner. Spray the nail, neon pink and yellow, as shown.

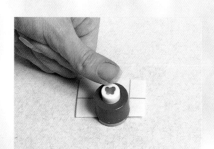

2 Cut out a large rectangle of "Frisket" film and place the butterfly on the plastic surface. Press down to engage the cutter.

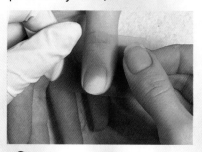

3 Peel the adhesive layer from the backing, and press it—adhesive-side down—on the nail. The base colors will be protected by the film.

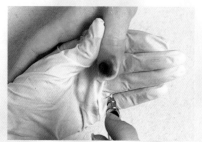

4 Spray the butterfly, black. Pass the airbrush swiftly over the stencil a number of times to make the butterfly stand out. Remove film.

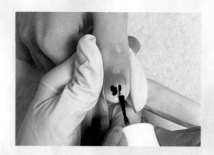

5 Apply coats of clear nail polish. Remove the overspray with soapy water and a cotton bud. Clean the airbrush following the manufacturer's instructions.

Chantilly lace

1. Apply a clear base coat, and allow to dry. Airbrush the nail white. Spray away excess paint (see page 89) with cleaner before each color change. Spray the nail with gold paint.

2. Hold the lace firmly over the nail, and spray with black paint. When dry, carefully lift off the lace.

3. Apply coats of clear polish. Remove the overspray with soapy water and cotton buds. Clean the airbrush following the manufacturer's instructions.

You will need: clear base coat; airbrush equipment and cleaner; white, gold, and black paint; piece of lace; clear nail polish; and cotton buds.

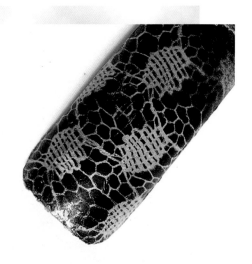

Chevron plus

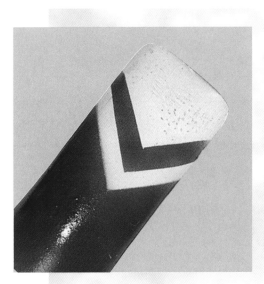

1. Apply a clear base coat, and allow to dry. Spray the nail white. Spray away excess paint (see page 89) with cleaner before each color change. Airbrush the nail, pink.

2. Hold the French chevron stencil firmly over the nail, leaving the nail tip area exposed. Spray the exposed nail with white paint. When dry, carefully remove the stencil.

3. Apply coats of clear polish. Remove the overspray with soapy water and cotton buds. Clean the airbrush following the manufacturer's instructions.

You will need: clear base coat, airbrush equipment and cleaner, white and pink paint, French chevron stencil, clear nail polish, and cotton buds.

Art deco

1. Apply a clear base coat, and allow to dry. Airbrush the nail white. Spray away excess paint (see page 89) with cleaner before each color change. Spray the nail with purple paint.

2. Select a stencil shape and position it firmly over the nail, and spray with your choice of color. Repeat to build up an interesting design, allowing the paint to dry before removing the stencils.

3. Apply coats of clear polish. Remove the overspray with soapy water and cotton buds. Clean the airbrush following the manufacturer's instructions.

You will need: clear base coat; airbrush equipment and cleaner; white, purple, green, yellow, blue, and gray paint; stencils; clear nail polish; and cotton buds.

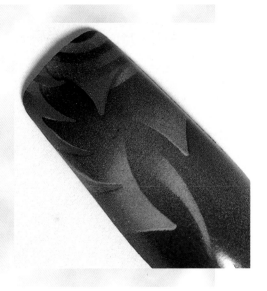

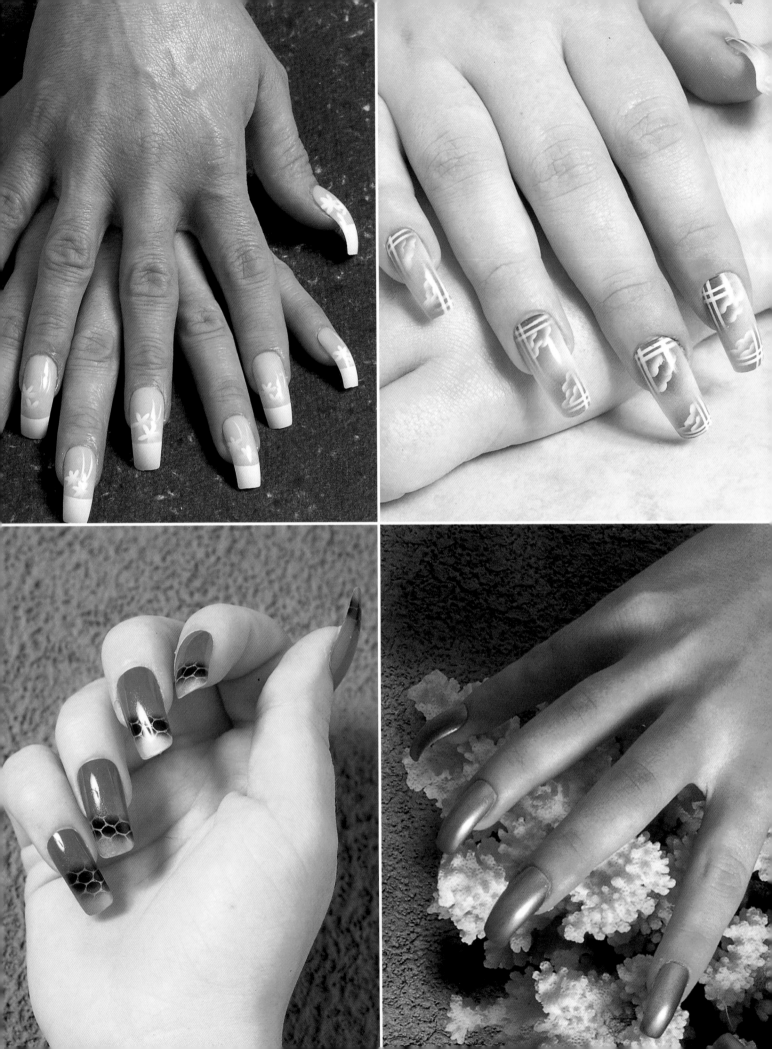

11

Nail Jewelry

Nail art and jewelry were made for each other. The results are spectacularly glamorous. There are so many different ways to achieve great effects, there's sure to be one that suits you.

Attaching jewelry to nails can be done in a number of different ways. The simplest method is to place a gold or silver charm, available from your nail art retailer, onto wet nail polish and then apply a top coat of clear varnish to keep it secure. To remove the charm, just apply nail polish remover.

At the other end of the spectrum is jewelry attached to the nail by a chain, clip, or tiny screw. If you want to go this route, remember you should not drill through natural nail since the nail can crack, and a hole in a natural nail will gradually wear and become larger. For these reasons drill holes only in nail extensions—they are easily drilled through—or first wrap your natural nail with acrylic or fiberglass.

A good sort of drill is a "Combi", a small metal device with a drill at one end and a socket at the other end for tightening the tiny nuts that hold on your charms.

To drill a hole, first clip the dangle onto the nail so you can get the right position for the hole. Too far from the edge and the dangle may not fit; too close and it may protrude over the tip.

When drilling, make sure you place the fingernail on a firm, but not solid, surface—a nail buffer or piece of cork are perfect. The hand must be palm up. Drill through the nail until the drill's tip starts to appear on the other side. Then slowly remove the drill, turn the hand palm down and gently push the drill tip into the hole from the top side. Buff the nail to smooth ridges around the hole.

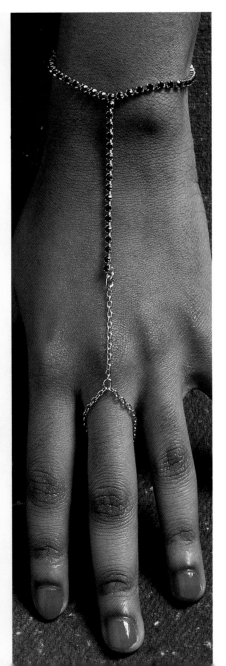

Posted charm

The posted charm is the most secure way of wearing precious gems on your nails. A posted charm can only be removed by undoing the nut. Before drilling, prepare the extended or acrylic-wrapped nail with a base coat, two coats of colored nail polish, and a coat of clear nail polish.

You will need:

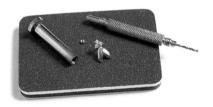

- base coat
- colored nail polish
- clear nail polish
- nail buffer or finger-rest
- Combi-type drill
- posted charm nail jewelry

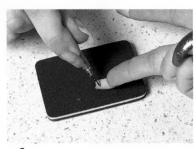

1 Position the drill tip 1/8th inch from the nail tip. Turn the drill to the right several times. When the tip strikes the buffer, slowly withdraw the drill.

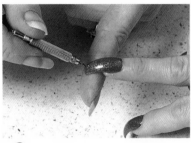

2 Turn the hand palm down, and gently push the drill tip into the hole to clear the hole. Buff the nail to smooth the hole, without damaging the nail polish.

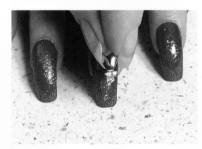

3 Push the screw of the posted charm through the hole from the top surface of the nail.

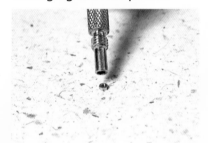

4 Push the socket-end of the drill over the nut. The nut will be held inside the socket opening. If not, moisten the socket-end by dabbing it onto a damp sponge first.

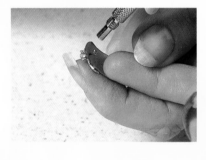

5 Place the socket-end of the drill onto the posted charm screw and start to turn the drill. This will screw the nut in place and secure the posted charm.

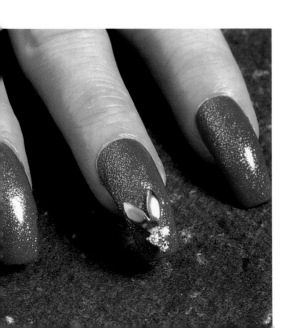

Clip-on ring chain

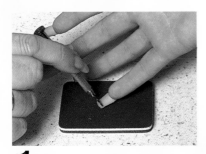

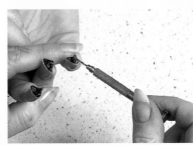

This piece of nail jewelry is best worn on a little finger for practical reasons. Prepare the extended or acrylic-wrapped nail with a base coat, two coats of colored nail polish, and a coat of clear nail polish.

1 Position the drill tip about 1/8th inch from the nail tip. Turn the drill to the right several times, until the tip strikes the buffer. Slowly withdraw the drill.

2 Turn the hand palm down. Gently push the drill tip into the hole to clear it. Carefully buff around the hole, without damaging the nail polish.

You will need:

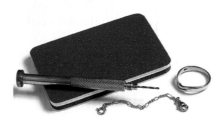

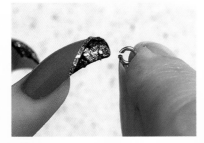

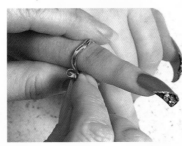

3 Pull down the trigger to open the clasp and attach it to the nail. Make sure the trigger is concealed on the underside of the nail and that the chain is the right length.

4 Place the ring onto the finger. Pull the trigger on the chain to open the clasp and attach it to the ring.

- base coat
- colored nail polish and design of your choice
- clear nail polish
- large nail buffer
- Combi-type drill
- ring chain clip-on jewelry

Hiding a mistake

If you drill a hole in the wrong place—too close to the tip or in the wrong position along the free edge—or decide you don't need the hole any more, it is easily rectified. Simply apply two coats of nail polish—clear or pigmented—all over the nail. The polish will fill the hole so that it is undetectable.

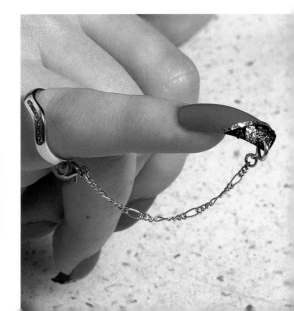

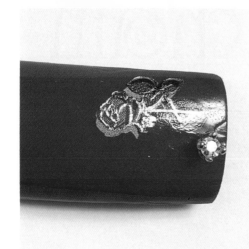

Diamond-tipped

1. Prepare the extended or acrylic-wrapped nail with a base coat, two coats of colored nail polish, and a coat of clear nail polish.

2. Using the same method as shown on page 98, drill a hole through the nail.

3. Very lightly buff the nail to smooth the surface around the hole. Using the socket-end of the drill to pick up the nut, turn the drill to screw the nut into place. Gently tighten to secure.

You will need: base coat, color nail polish, clear nail polish, large nail buffer, "Combi" type drill, and a posted charm stud.

Ring and ball

1. Prepare the extended or wrapped nail with a base coat, coats of colored nail polish, and a coat of clear nail polish. Use the method on page 98 to drill a hole along the free edge. Buff to smooth the hole.

2. Pick up the ring with tweezers, each holding onto one side of the join. The join should be uppermost. To open the join: pull back with one pair of tweezers, push forward with the other.

3. Hold the ring with one pair of tweezers, and use the other to slide the ball onto the ring. Pass the ring through the hole from underneath the tip. Use both pairs of tweezers to close the ring.

You will need: base coat, color nail polish, clear polish, nail buffer, "Combi" type drill, ring and ball jewelry, and 2 pairs of tweezers.

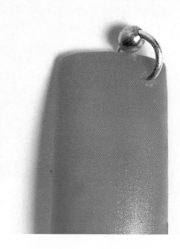

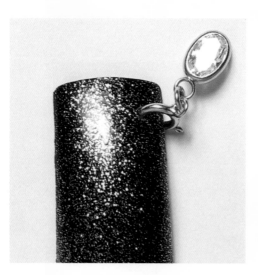

Dangle

1. Prepare the extended or acrylic-wrapped nail with a base coat, two coats of colored nail polish, and a coat of clear nail polish.

2. Use the method as shown on page 98 to drill a hole a little down one edge of the nail tip. Very lightly buff the nail to smooth the surface around the hole, but without damaging the nail polish.

3. Pull back on the trigger to open the clasp on the ring. Clip the ring into the hole with the clasp hidden under the nail tip.

You will need: base coat, color nail polish, clear nail polish, large nail buffer, "Combi" type drill, and clip-on dangle jewelry.

Goldfinger

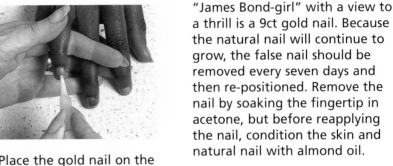

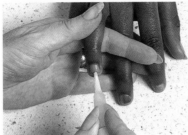

1 Thoroughly clean the natural nail to remove polish and oil film with nail polish remover.

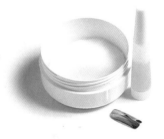

2 Place the gold nail on the natural nail and check for fit. It may be necessary to gently file the edges, but take great care not to scratch the gold surface. Apply a small amount of nail adhesive down the length of the natural nail. Note: the glue dries very quickly.

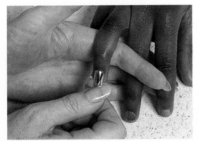

3 Position, at an angle, the end of the gold nail into the cuticle area. Slowly lower it onto the natural nail and hold it in place for a few seconds. Wipe off any excess glue with a cotton bud dipped in acetone. Clean the gold nail with a jewelry cleaner, and be scrupulous about hygiene behind the nail tip.

The ultimate for any aspiring "James Bond-girl" with a view to a thrill is a 9ct gold nail. Because the natural nail will continue to grow, the false nail should be removed every seven days and then re-positioned. Remove the nail by soaking the fingertip in acetone, but before reapplying the nail, condition the skin and natural nail with almond oil.

You will need:

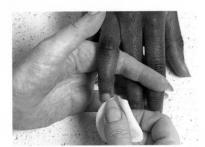

- acetone-free nail polish remover
- 9ct gold nail
- nail adhesive glue (strong and fast-drying)

Quality products

The range of nail art equipment, cosmetics, and decorations increases daily. And because the choice is so dazzling, it is even more important that you take the time to buy quality products that will do no damage to your natural nails. If in doubt, always seek the advice of a qualified nail technician.

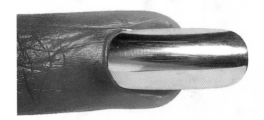

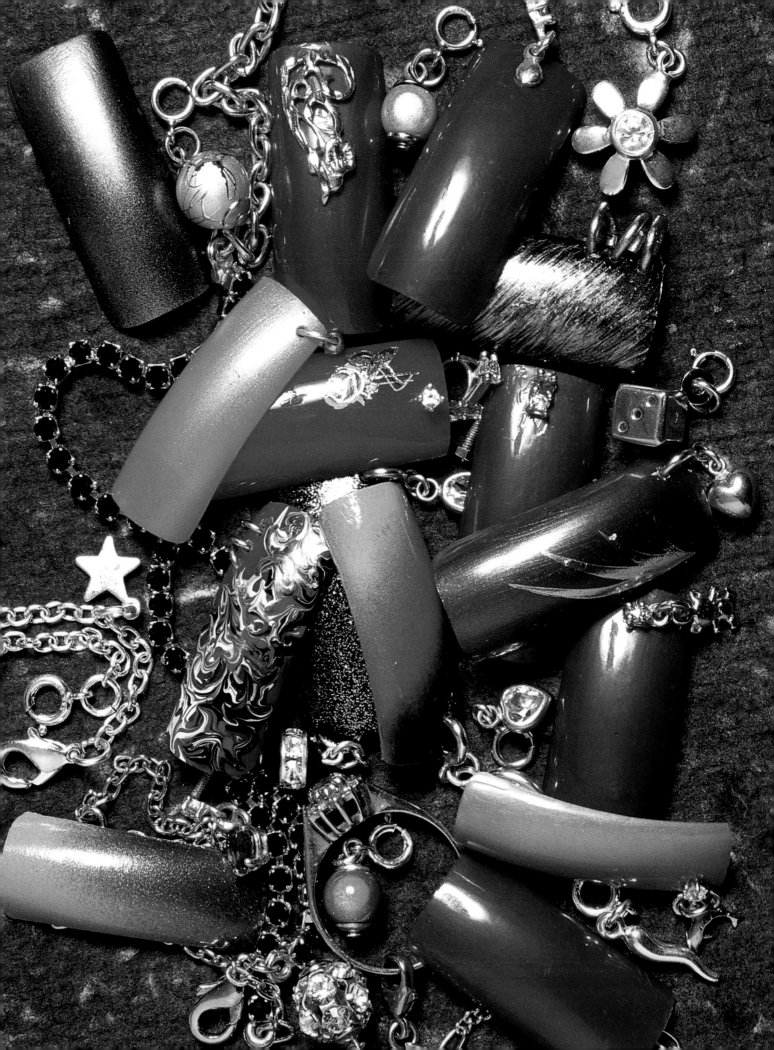

12

Pure Fantasy

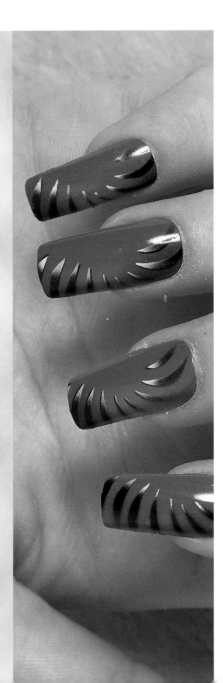

There is absolutely nothing practical about these fantasy designs. When wearing them, forget about doing anything except posing.

These creations show just how far nail art has developed from it's humble beginnings. Professional nail artists do in miniature what canvas artists and fashion gurus do on a human scale. Size is no drawback to the nail artist wishing to express her or himself. And evidence of their skill and boundless imagination is reflected by their status in the world of cutting-edge styling for the catwalk models and high-fashion photography. Other than a "Protrans" kit

(there are other transfer kits on the market, but the instructions in this book relate only to "Protrans"), and acrylic liquid and powder—both available from nail art suppliers—fantasy nail art does not rely on gadgets or equipment. Everything you really need, you've already got—imagination, a sense of humour, and a willingness to endure the trial and error process until you achieve the results you desire. Go on and have a try, there's nothing but fun to be had.

Pop-out goldfish

Though not the work of a moment, this nail art underwater scene and three-dimensional fish will have people stopping you in the street. It is just that amazing!

You will need:

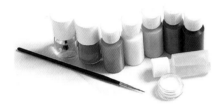

- base coat
- blue nail polish
- acrylic liquid and powder
- fine-tip brush suitable for acrylics
- sheet of flexible plastic
- orange, light and dark green, white, and black paint
- fine-tip art brush
- clear nail varnish

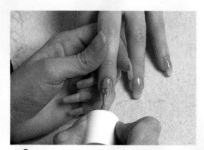

1 Apply a base coat and two coats of blue nail polish, and allow to dry.

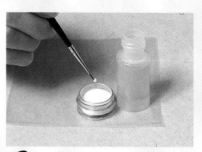

2 Mix together, following the manufacturer's instructions, the acrylic liquid and powder to form a ball on the end of the acrylic brush.

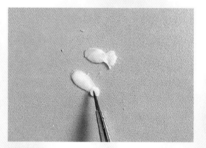

3 Place the ball of acrylic onto the plastic and mould it in to the fish's body. Mould a smaller ball of acrylic to make the tail. Make two fish. Put aside to dry.

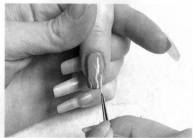

4 Put small amounts of each paint onto a palette. Using the art brush and green paints, paint the reeds.

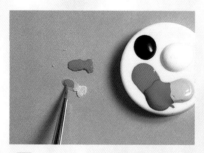

5 When the acrylic is dry, paint the fish orange. Put dots of "wet" acrylic onto the nail where you want to position the fish.

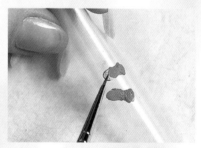

6 Bend the plastic and lift off the fish using the brush. Press them into place on the nail. Finish painting the scene, then apply two coats of clear nail polish.

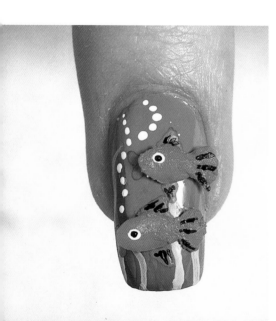

Clever fakes

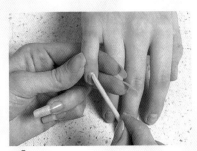

1 Remove any nail polish and greasy film from the natural nail with polish remover. Gently push back the cuticle.

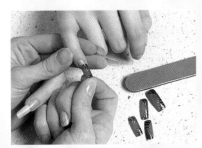

2 Place the fake nail on the natural nail and check the fit. File, if necessary, taking care not to damage the finish on colored or decorated stick-ons.

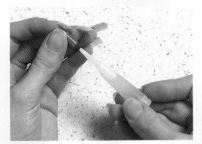

3 Pierce the container of nail glue with the pin concealed inside the top of the lid. Apply a small amount of glue in a line down the length of the natural nail.

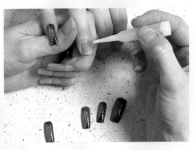

4 Holding the stick-on nail by the tip and at a slight angle, place the end into the cuticle area of the natural nail. Slowly lower the nail onto the natural nail. Hold in place until the glue dries. Wipe off any excess glue.

Whether you use stick-on nails just for a "big night out" or to temporarily conceal a broken nail, they have come into their own in the last few years. Improvements have lead to a more natural look and better fit. Stick-on nails come in many styles—plain, colored or decorated—and in different lengths from practical and sporty to the downright dangerous!

You will need:

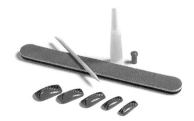

- orangewood stick
- acetone-free nail polish remover
- emery board
- stick-on nails of your choice
- nail adhesive glue

Kindness counts

Be kind to your natural nails by wearing stick-on nails for no longer than five days. Remove the stick-ons, following a nail technician's advice or the instructions on the nail kit, and then treat your natural nails to a full manicure and moisturizing and conditioning treatment. Never try to simply tear stick-on nails off—it will damage the nail plate.

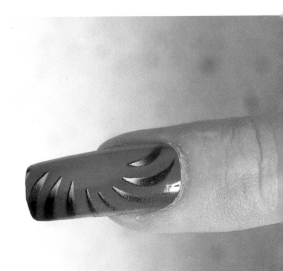

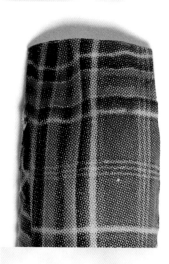

Clan tartan

1. Choose a frame from the "Protrans" kit that matches the nail to be decorated. Place the frame over your chosen picture. Cut out the picture slightly larger than the frame.

2. Apply a coat of Transfixer onto the front of the picture. When dry, the Transfixer becomes a clear film. Saturate the back of the picture with water. Use the harsh surface of the peeling block to score the back of the picture. Then use the soft surface to remove the paper. You will be left with a transparent "transfer".

3. Apply a base coat and white nail polish to the nail. When dry, press and smooth the "transfer" onto the nail. Cut off any excess transfer, before coating with clear nail polish.

You will need: magazine picture or a photocopy of a photograph, "Protrans" kit, base coat, white nail polish, and clear nail varnish.

Nail feathers

1. Apply a base coat and coats of white nail polish, and allow to dry. Paint half of the nail pink using the liner brush. Make the edge jagged where the pink meets the white polish.

2. Secure the feathers along the jagged line, using the glue. Paint the nail and the end tips of the feathers with clear nail polish.

3. While the clear polish is wet, position polish-secure decorations. Use decorations to conceal the end tips of the feathers. Finish with another coat of clear nail varnish.

You will need: base coat, white nail polish, neon pink acrylic paint, liner brush, low-strength nail glue, feathers, clear nail polish, tweezers, and polish-secure decorations.

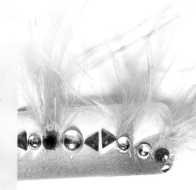

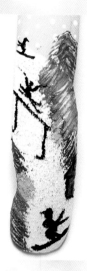

Skiing, anyone?

1. After "building" the fake nail, file the edges to form the curves. Mix together the acrylic powder and liquid (see page 104) and paint it over the nail. When dry, smooth with a buffer. Secure the nail to the natural nail following the instructions on page 105.

2. Apply a base coat and a coat of blue polish, and allow to dry. Paint the ski run white and, while wet, sprinkle over the glitter.

3. Use the paints and art brush to complete the scene. When dry, apply a coat of clear varnish.

You will need: extra-long stick-on nail or three shorter ones glued end-to-end; acrylic liquid and powder, and brush; nail buffer; nail glue; base coat; blue polish; pearl glitter; fine-tip art brush; white, green, brown, and black acrylic paints; and clear nail polish.

Cut above

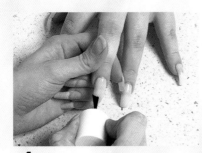

1 Apply a base coat to the nail extension. Cut-outs can be done on stick-on nails before they are fixed to your natural nails.

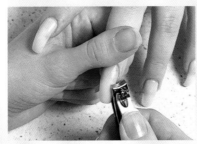

2 Use the nail clippers to make a small, "V" shaped cut into one side edge.

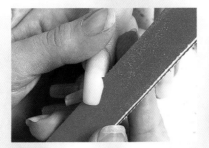

3 File any rough edges. Make a "V" shaped cut on the other side edge. File to smooth edges.

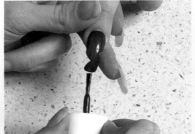

4 Apply a second base coat before painting the nail with two coats of blue polish.

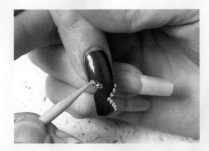

5 While the final coat of polish is wet, position rhinestones along the cut edges. Should the polish dry, apply a coat of clear polish and continue. Finish with a coat of clear nail polish.

There's is no end to what you can do–as long as you're wearing nail extensions. Don't even think about doing this to your natural nails because they will never forgive you.

You will need:

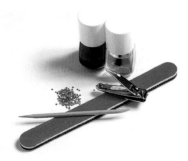

- base coat
- small nail clippers
- emery board
- blue nail polish
- rhinestones
- orangewood stick
- clear nail polish

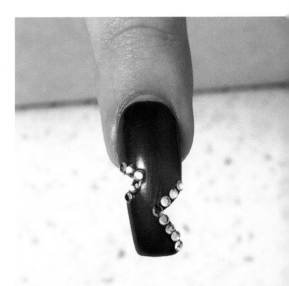

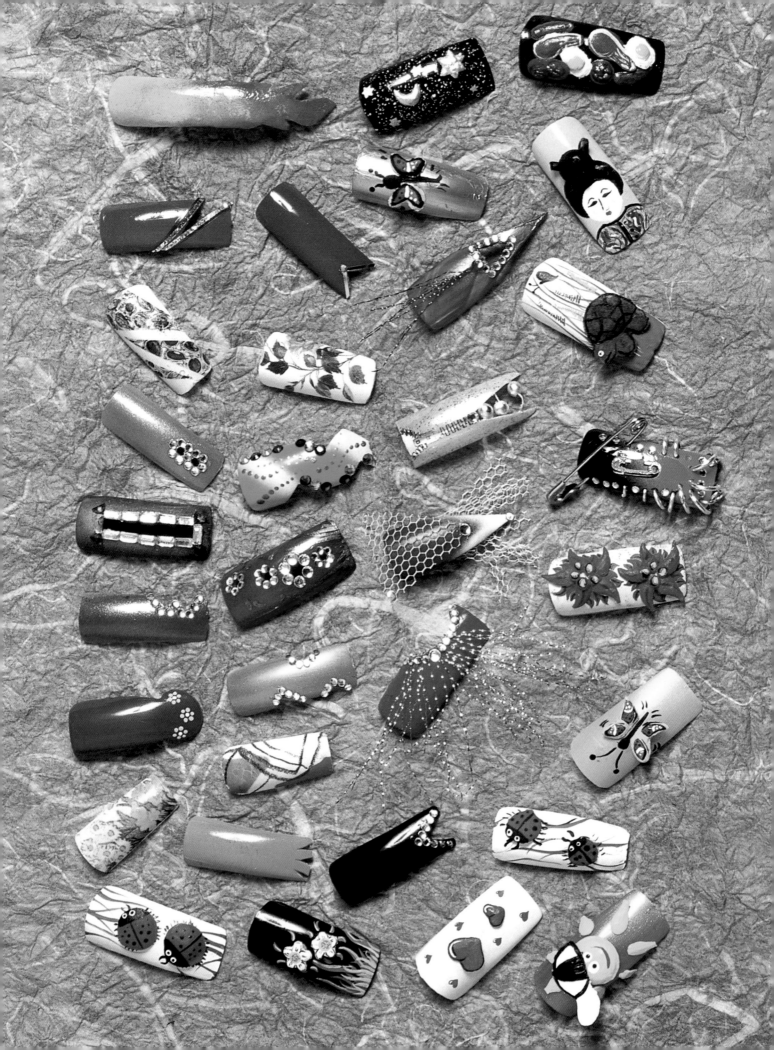

Index

A

Abstract designs 28, 31, 39, 50, 51, 52, 58, 71, 82, 83, 87, 92, 95
Acetone 16
Acrylic modelling 104, 106
Acrylic nail paint 12, 57, 65
    designs 55, 66-72
Airbrush designs 89-96
    cleaning 89
    equipment 12, 89
    gallery 93, 96
    lace 12
    paint 12
All-over design 58
American chevron 43
American design 41
"Angle-chisel" tool 12
Animal designs 28, 30, 31, 37, 38, 55, 59, 60, 71, 74, 79, 91, 94, 104
Art brushes 12
Art deco 95
Arty nail 39

B

Balloon's away 62
Bands of gold 55
Base coat 12
Be-dazzled 23
Biotin 10
Body painting 8
Bow 63
Brittle nails 10
Bruising 10
Brushes
    art 12
    fan 12
    sable glitter dust 13
    stripping 13
Brushstrokes 87
Buffing 14
Butterfly 55

C

Calcium 10
Carnival 84
C-curve 41
Chantilly lace 95
Charms
    polish-secure 20
Cherries 53
Chevron designs 43, 44, 44, 52, 84, 95
Chevron foil 84
Chevron of pearls 44
Chevron plus 95
Children's designs 19, 20, 23, 28, 41, 47, 58, 60 62, 63, 68, 71, 74, 76, 78, 79, 94
Chinese character 76
Clan tartan 106
Clever fakes 105
Clip-on ring chain 99
Clowning around 19
"Color Shaper" tools 12, 65
Confetti 68
Craft knife 12
Creams
    feet 15
    hand 11, 14
    nail 11, 14
"Cup-round" tool 12
Cut above 107
Cuticle
    nippers 14, 15
    conditioning cream 11
    care 14, 16
    remover 11
Cutter punch 12

D

Dab-a-doo 68
Daisy chain 47
Dangle 100
"Dazzell" designs 23
Decals 12, 33-40
    method 33
Dents 10
Diamond-crystal designs 20, 21, 30, 51
Diamond snake 30
Diamonds and glitter 20
Diamonds are forever 51
Diamond-tipped 100
Diet 10
Dolphin watch 79
Duo-tone 92

E

Embossed designs 57-64
    method 57
    gallery 61, 64
Embossing
    paint 12, 57
    strokes 57
    tool 12, 57
Emery boards 11
    manicure 14, 15
Eye of the tiger 91

F

Fan brush 12, 65
Fanfare 70
Fantasy designs
    see Pure fantasy
Flaking 10
Flatstone designs 23, 47
Food designs 53, 60
Floral designs 18, 35, 36, 38, 44, 47, 52, 63, 78, 86
Floral bouquet 35
Flower power 78
Foil leafing 12
    polish-secure 22
Foil designs 81-88
    gallery 85, 88
    method 81
Foil flower 86
Foils 12
French chevron 44
French designs 41-48, 52
    gallery 45, 48
    guide tapes 12
    method 41

French polish 42
French manicure
    see French designs
French transfer 44
Frisket butterfly 94
Frisket film 12, 89
From A to Z 76

G

Geometric designs 26, 27, 28, 55, 62, 92
Gilded roses 39
Glitter dust 12, 49-56
    brush 12
    gallery 53, 56
    method 49
Glittering chevron 52
Glitter tipped 47
Go geometric 28
Going dotty 71
Goldfinger 101
Goo-goo eyes 19
Guide tapes 12, 41

H

Habitat designs 34, 36, 74, 79, 92, 106
Half and half 84
Hand-painted designs 73-80, 104, 106
    gallery 77, 80
Hardeners 11
Henna 6
History 6
Holiday designs 36, 60, 62, 63, 68, 74, 79, 84, 87, 106

I

Indian aum 76
Iodine 10
It's a gas 67

J

Jewel finish 28
Jewelry
    see Nail jewelry
Jungle beat 92

L

Lace
    designs 36, 46, 95
    fabric 12
Lace netting 36
Lettering 76
Leopard spots 71
Liner brush 12, 65
Line up 27

M

Marbling
    designs 66,
    tool 12
Massage
    foot 15
    hand 15
Mendhi 8
Mirage 83

N

Nail adhesive glue 12
    solvent 16
Nail art
    equipment 12-13
    removal 16
    sealer 12
Nail buffer 11
Nail feathers 106
Nail manicure 14
    equipment 11
Nail extensions 9, 11
    removal 16
Nail
    health 10, 11, 13, 14, 16

cutting 14, 15
Nail jewelry designs 97-102
    attaching 102
    gallery 102
    types 12, 102
Nail paints
    see Acrylic nail paints
Nail polish
    applying 14
    care 8
    colors 8
    quality 8
    remover 11, 16
    thinners 11
Nail scissors 11
Nail shape 8
Nail technician 10
Neon shower 52
New York, New York 79

O

Oils 11
On the Prowl 38
Opalescent paint, 23, 65
    Orangewood sticks 12

P

Paint and polish 65-72
    gallery 68, 72
    paint 12, 65
    tools 12, 13
Palm d'Or 87
Palm tree 75
Parrot fashion 74
Paws for thought 60
Pearl designs 23, 44
Pearl drops 23
Pedicure 15
Polish-secure designs 17-24, 30, 44, 47, 52, 55, 106
    gallery 21, 25
    method 17
    removal 16
Polka dots 82
Pop-out goldfish 104
Post and charm jewelry 98, 100
Posted charm 98
"Protrans" 103, 105
Pure fantasy 103-109

Quick-drying sealer 11

Racy stripes 63
Rhinestone flower 18
Rhinestone designs 18, 19, 47, 52, 55, 84, 107
Rhinestone diamond 55
Ring and ball 100
Ring chain 99
Rose tips 36

Sable glitter dust brush 12
Self-adhesive decorations 25-32
Shock waves 68
Silver shield 87
Simply charming 20
Skiing, anyone? 106
Skinned and striped 31
"Smile" line 41
Snakes alive 39
Snakeskin designs 28, 30, 31, 38

Snowdrop 63
Sparkle nail polish 21
Split image 84
Splitting 10
Spooky 60
Stained glass 50
Staining 10
Stencils 13, 65, 91, 92, 94, 95
Stick-on
    art 13, 25-32
    gallery 29, 32
    nails 11, 13, 101, 105, 106
    removal 16
Strawberry sundae 60
Strengtheners 11
Stripes on parade 26
Striping brush 13, 65
Striping tape designs 26, 27, 28, 30, 31, 47, 87,
Stop 'n' go 79
Stud designs 20
Stud work 20
Sulfur 10
Swanning around 59
Sweetheart bow 63
Swirl time 31

"Taper-point" tool 12
Tiger, tiger 71
Top coat 11, 12
Totally abstract 92

Touch of lace 46
Transfers 12, 33-40
    French 41, 44, 46
    gallery 37, 40
    method 33
Tri-tone 90
Tropical daze 36
Tweezers 12

Valentine hearts 31
Vertical grooves 10
Vitamin A 10
Vitamin B 10
Vive la difference 47

Wedding designs 18, 20, 23, 35, 36, 36, 38, 42, 43, 44, 52, 76 47, 99
    Weak nails 10
White marks 10
White nail pencil 11
Wild thing 34

Acknowledgements

The authors would like to thank the K-Sa-Ra team, Kirsty, Sarah, Tina, and Louise.
Special thanks to Sue Hammond for her design ideas and encouragement.
The editor would like to thank Lynn Langendoen of "Fingertips", Hampshire for all her help and advice.
Thanks to the K-Sa-Ra suppliers, and also the models, Ananta, Charlie, Zoe, Rob, Ade, Jenny, Camphan and Monique.